D0989325

*Quick*FACTS™

Thyroid
CANCER

What You Need to Know—NOW

Kirtland Community College Library
10775 N. St. Helen Rd.
Roscommon, MI 48653
989.275.5000 x 246

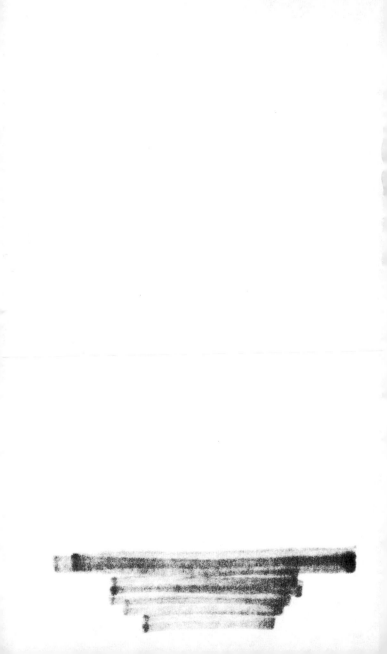

*Quick*FACTS™

From the Experts at the American Cancer Society

Thyroid
CANCER

What You Need to Know—NOW

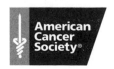

Published by the American Cancer Society/Health Promotions
250 Williams Street NW, Atlanta, Georgia 30303 USA

Copyright ©2009 American Cancer Society

All rights reserved. Without limiting the rights under copyright
reserved above, no part of this publication may be reproduced,
stored in or introduced into a retrieval system, or transmitted
in any form or by any means (electronic, mechanical, photo-
copying, recording, or otherwise) without the prior written
permission of the publisher.

Printed in the United States of America
Cover designed by Jill Dible, Atlanta, GA
Edited by Vivian Farah McGee, Raleigh, NC
Composition by Graphic Composition, Inc.

5 4 3 2 1   09 10 11 12 13

Library of Congress Cataloging-in-Publication Data

Quickfacts thyroid cancer: what you need to know now.
    p. cm. — (Quickfacts)
  Includes bibliographical references and index.
  ISBN-13: 978-0-944235-82-9 (pbk : alk. paper)
  ISBN-10: 0-944235-82-4 (pbk : alk. paper)
  1. Thyroid gland—Cancer—Popular works. I. American
Cancer Society.
RC280.T6Q53 2009
616.99'444–dc22

                                        2008042607

A Note to the Reader

This information represents the views of the doctors and nurses
serving on the American Cancer Society's Cancer Information
Database Editorial Board. These views are based on their
interpretation of studies published in medical journals, as well
as their own professional experience.

The treatment information in this book is not official policy of
the Society and is not intended as medical advice to replace the
expertise and judgment of your cancer care team. It is intended
to help you and your family make informed decisions, together
with your doctor.

Your doctor may have reasons for suggesting a treatment plan
different from these general treatment options. Don't hesitate to
ask him or her questions about your treatment options.

For more information, contact your American Cancer Society
at **800-ACS-2345** or **http://www.cancer.org**.

Bulk purchases of this book are available at a discount.
For information, contact the American Cancer Society at
trade.sales@cancer.org.

For special sales, contact us at **trade.sales@cancer.org**.

TABLE OF CONTENTS

Treatment

Questions to Ask

After Treatment

Latest Research

What's New in Thyroid Cancer Research and Treatment? 91

Resources 95

Glossary 99

Index 121

Your Thyroid Cancer

What Is Cancer?

Cancer* develops when cells in a part of the body begin to grow out of control. Although there are many kinds of cancer, they all start because of out-of-control growth of abnormal cells.

Normal body cells grow, divide, and die in an orderly fashion. During the early years of a person's life, normal cells divide rapidly. Then, after a person becomes an adult, cells in most parts of the body divide only to replace worn-out or dying cells and to repair injuries.

Because **cancer cells** continue to grow and divide, they are different from normal cells. Instead of dying like normal cells do, they continue to form new abnormal cells.

Cancer cells develop because of damage to **DNA.** DNA is in every cell and directs all of a cell's activities. Most of the time when DNA becomes damaged, the body is able to repair it. In cancer cells, the damaged DNA is not repaired. People can inherit damaged DNA, which accounts for

*Terms in **bold type** are further explained in the Glossary, beginning on page 99.*

inherited cancers. Many times though, a person's DNA becomes damaged by exposure to something in the environment, like smoke.

Cancer usually forms as a **tumor.** Some cancers, like leukemia, do not form tumors. Instead, these cancer cells involve the blood and blood-forming organs, such as bone marrow, and circulate through other **tissues** where they grow. Often, cancer cells travel to other parts of the body where they begin to grow and replace normal tissue. This process is called **metastasis.** Regardless of where a cancer may spread, it is always named for the place it began. For instance, breast cancer that spreads to the liver is still called breast cancer, not liver cancer. Not all tumors are cancerous. Benign (noncancerous) tumors do not spread (**metastasize**) to other parts of the body and, with very rare exceptions, are not life threatening.

Different types of cancer can behave very differently. For example, lung cancer and breast cancer are very different diseases. They grow at different rates and respond to different treatments. Therefore, people with cancer need treatment that is aimed at their particular kind of cancer.

Cancer is the second leading cause of death in the United States. Cancer will develop in nearly half of all men and in a little over one third of all women in the United States during their lifetimes. Today, millions of people are living with cancer or have had cancer. The risk for developing most types of cancer can be reduced by changes in a person's lifestyle, for example, by quitting smoking and eating a healthier diet. The sooner a cancer is found and treatment begun, the better are a person's chances for living many years.

What Is Thyroid Cancer?

Thyroid cancer is a cancer that starts in the **thyroid gland.** In order to understand thyroid cancer, it helps to know about the normal structure and function of the thyroid gland. The thyroid gland is located under the Adam's apple in the front part of the neck. In most people, it cannot be seen or felt. It is butterfly-shaped, with 2 **lobes**—the right lobe and the left lobe—joined by a narrow isthmus (see picture below).

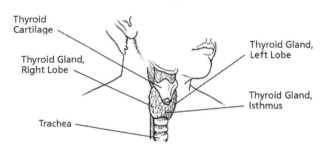

The thyroid gland contains 2 main types of cells: **thyroid follicular cells** and **C cells** (also called **parafollicular cells**).

The follicular cells use **iodine** from the blood to make thyroid hormone, which helps regulate a person's **metabolism.** Too much thyroid hormone (called **hyperthyroidism**) can cause a rapid or irregular heartbeat, sleep problems, nervousness, hunger, weight loss, and a feeling of being too warm. Too little hormone (called **hypothyroidism**) can cause a person to slow down, feel tired, and gain weight. The amount of thyroid hormone released by the thyroid is regulated by the **pituitary gland,** which is at the base of the brain and makes a substance called **thyroid-stimulating hormone (TSH).**

C cells (parafollicular cells) make **calcitonin,** a hormone that helps regulate how the body uses calcium.

Other less common cells in the thyroid gland include immune system cells (**lymphocytes**) and supportive (**stromal**) **cells.**

Different cancers develop from each kind of cell. These differences are important because they affect the patient's outlook for survival and what type of treatment is needed.

Most tumors that develop in the thyroid gland are **benign** (noncancerous). Others are **malignant** (cancerous), which means they can spread into nearby tissues and to other parts of the body.

Benign Thyroid Enlargement and Nodules

Because the thyroid gland is right under the skin, changes in its size and shape can often be felt or even seen by patients or by their doctor.

The medical term for an abnormally large thyroid gland is a **goiter.** Some goiters are diffuse, meaning that the whole gland is large. Other goiters are nodular, meaning that the gland is large and has one or more bumps in it. There are many reasons the thyroid gland might be larger than usual, and most of the time it is not cancer. Both diffuse and nodular goiters are usually caused by an imbalance in certain hormones; for example, not getting enough iodine in the diet can cause changes in hormone levels and lead to a goiter.

Lumps or bumps in the thyroid gland are called **thyroid nodules.** Most thyroid nodules are benign, but about 1 in 20 is cancerous (see "Malignant Thyroid Tumors" on page 6).

Thyroid nodules can develop in people of all ages, but they are most common in older adults. Fewer than 1 in 10 adults have thyroid nodules that can be felt by a doctor. When tested with ultrasound scanning of the thyroid gland, up to half of all people are found to have nodules that are too small to feel.

Most nodules are **cysts** filled with fluid or with a stored form of thyroid hormone called **colloid.** A colloid nodule is one of the most common types of thyroid nodules.

Solid nodules have little fluid or colloid. Some solid nodules may have too many cells, but the cells are not cancer cells. These types of nodules include **hyperplastic** nodules and **adenomas.** Sometimes these nodules make too much thyroid hormone and cause hyperthyroidism. Thyroid nodules that have been found to be benign can sometimes be left alone (instead of being treated) as long as they're not growing or causing symptoms. Others may require some form of treatment.

Malignant Thyroid Tumors

Only about 1 in 20 thyroid nodules is cancerous. The 2 most common types of thyroid cancer are called **papillary carcinoma** and **follicular carcinoma. Hürthle cell carcinoma** is a subtype of follicular carcinoma. There are some other types of thyroid cancer that occur less frequently, including **medullary thyroid carcinoma (MTC), anaplastic carcinoma, thyroid lymphoma,** and **thyroid sarcoma.**

Papillary Carcinoma

Most thyroid cancers—about 8 of 10—are papillary carcinomas (also called **papillary thyroid cancers** or **papillary adenocarcinomas**). Papillary carcinomas typically grow very slowly. Usually, they develop in only one lobe of the thyroid gland, but sometimes they occur in both lobes. Even though they grow slowly, papillary carcinomas often spread to the **lymph nodes** in the neck. But most of the time, this **regional metastasis** can be successfully treated and is rarely fatal.

Several different variants (subtypes) of papillary carcinoma can be recognized under the microscope. Of these, the follicular variant occurs most often. The usual form of papillary carcinoma and the follicular variant have the same outlook for survival (**prognosis**), and treatment is the same for both. Other variants of papillary carcinoma (columnar, tall cell, diffuse sclerosis) are not as common and tend to grow and spread more quickly.

Follicular Carcinoma

Follicular carcinoma, also called **follicular thyroid cancer** or **follicular adenocarcinoma,** is the next most common type of thyroid cancer. Follicular cancer is much less common than papillary thyroid cancer, occurring in 1 of 10 thyroid cancers. It is more common in countries where people don't get enough iodine in their diet. Follicular cancer usually remains in the thyroid gland. Unlike papillary carcinoma, follicular carcinoma usually does not spread to lymph nodes, but it can spread to other parts of the body, such as the lungs or bones. The prognosis for follicular carcinoma is not quite as good as that for papillary carcinoma, although it is still very good in most cases.

Hürthle cell carcinoma, also known as **oxyphil cell carcinoma,** is a type of follicular carcinoma and accounts for about 4% of thyroid cancers. Hürthle cell carcinoma does not absorb radioactive iodine well. Therefore, it is harder to find and treat. The prognosis for Hürthle cell carcinoma may not be as good as that for typical follicular carcinoma.

Differentiated Thyroid Cancers

Differentiated thyroid cancers develop from thyroid follicular cells. The cells of differentiated thyroid cancers appear similar to those of normal thyroid tissue when examined under a microscope. In cancer, differentiation refers to how mature (developed) the cancer cells are in a tumor. Differentiated tumor cells tend to grow and spread more slowly than undifferentiated (or poorly differentiated) tumor cells, which lack the structure and function of normal cells and grow uncontrollably. Undifferentiated cancer is sometimes referred to as an anaplastic cancer.

Other Types of Thyroid Cancers

Medullary thyroid carcinoma: Medullary thyroid carcinoma (MTC) accounts for about 5% of thyroid cancers. It develops from the C cells of the thyroid gland. Sometimes this cancer can spread to lymph nodes, the lungs, or liver even before a thyroid nodule is discovered or a screening test is done. These cancers usually make calcitonin and **carcinoembryonic antigen** (**CEA**), which can be found by blood tests. Calcitonin is a hormone that helps control the amount of calcium in the blood. CEA is a protein made by certain cancers, such as colorectal cancer and MTC. Because medullary cancer does not absorb or take up radioactive iodine (used for treatment and to find metastases), the prognosis (outlook) is not quite as good as that for differentiated thyroid cancers.

There are 2 types of MTC. The first type, occurring in about 8 out of 10 cases, is called **sporadic MTC.** The sporadic type is not inherited; that is, it does not run in families. It occurs mostly in older adults and in only one thyroid lobe. The other type of MTC is inherited and can occur in each generation of a family. This **familial MTC** often develops during childhood or early adulthood and can spread early. Familial MTC is often linked to an increased risk for other types of tumors. For more information, see the section "What Are the Risk Factors for Thyroid Cancer?" on page 13.

Anaplastic carcinoma: Anaplastic carcinoma (also called undifferentiated carcinoma) is a rare form of thyroid cancer, making up about 2% of all thyroid cancers. It is believed to develop from an existing papillary or follicular cancer. This cancer is called undifferentiated because the cancer cells lack the structure and function of normal cells; they do not look like normal thyroid tissue cells under the microscope. Anaplastic carcinoma is an aggressive cancer that rapidly invades the neck, often spreads to other parts of the body, and is very hard to treat.

Thyroid lymphoma: Lymphoma is uncommon in the thyroid gland. Lymphomas are cancers that develop from lymphocytes, the main cell type of the immune system. Most lymphocytes are found in lymph nodes, which are pea-sized collections of immune cells scattered throughout the body (including the thyroid gland).

Lymphomas are discussed in the American Cancer Society document *Non-Hodgkin Lymphoma,* available on the Web at **www.cancer.org** or by calling **800-ACS-2345.**

Thyroid sarcoma: Thyroid sarcomas are rare cancers that start in the supporting cells of the thyroid. They are often aggressive and hard to treat.

Sarcomas are discussed in the American Cancer Society document *Sarcoma: Adult Soft Tissue Cancer,* available on the Web at **www.cancer.org** or by calling **800-ACS-2345.**

Parathyroid Cancer

Attached behind the thyroid gland are 4 tiny glands called the **parathyroid glands.** The parathyroid glands help regulate the body's calcium levels. Cancers of the parathyroid glands are very rare—there are probably fewer than 100 cases each year in the United States. Parathyroid cancers cause the blood calcium levels to be elevated and lead to tiredness, weakness, and drowsiness. High blood calcium levels also cause frequent urination, which leads to dehydration and can worsen weakness and drowsiness.

Parathyroid cancer may also be detected as a thyroid nodule if it grows too large. No matter how large the nodule is, the only treatment is to remove it surgically. Unfortunately, parathyroid cancer is much harder to cure than thyroid cancer. The remainder of this book discusses only thyroid cancer.

What Are the Key Statistics About Thyroid Cancer?

The American Cancer Society estimated that about 37,340 new cases of thyroid cancer would be diagnosed in the United States in 2008—29,480 cases were attributed to women, and 8,930 to men. In general, thyroid cancer is one of the least deadly cancers. The **five (5)-year survival rate** (the percentage of people living *at least* 5 years after being diagnosed) for all cases is about 97%. (Statistics on survival rates by type and stage of thyroid cancer are discussed in the section, "How Is Thyroid

Cancer Staged?" on page 33.) Estimates for 2008 predicted that 910 women and 680 men (1,590 total) would die of thyroid cancer during the year. Thyroid cancer is different from many other adult cancers in that it primarily affects younger people. Nearly 2 of 3 cases occur in people between the ages of 20 and 55.

The chance of having thyroid cancer has risen slightly in recent years. Most of this increase in incidence is attributed to better diagnostic methods, that is, an increased use of thyroid **ultrasound,** which detects small thyroid nodules that might not otherwise have been found. Primarily, more small papillary cancers are being found, and these cancers are rarely fatal. The death rate from thyroid cancer has been fairly stable for many years.

Risk Factors and Causes

What Are the Risk Factors for Thyroid Cancer?

A **risk factor** is anything that affects a person's chance of getting a disease such as cancer. Different cancers have different risk factors. For example, exposing skin to strong sunlight is a risk factor for skin cancer. Smoking is a risk factor for a number of cancers. Risk factors don't tell us everything. Having a risk factor, or even several risk factors, does not mean that you will get the disease. Many people who get the disease may not have had any known risk factors. Even if a person with thyroid cancer has a risk factor, it is very hard to know how much that risk factor may have contributed to the cancer. Scientists have found a few risk factors that make cancer more likely to develop in the thyroid.

Gender and Age

For unclear reasons, thyroid cancers occur about 3 times more often in women than in men. Thyroid cancers can occur in people of all ages, but most cases of papillary and follicular thyroid cancers are found in people who are between 20 and 60 years of age.

Diet Low in Iodine

Follicular thyroid cancers are more common in areas of the world where people's diets are low in iodine. In the United States, dietary iodine is plentiful because iodine is added to table salt and other foods. A diet low in iodine may also increase the risk of papillary cancer if the person also is exposed to **radiation.**

Radiation

Exposure to radiation is a proven risk factor for thyroid cancer. Sources of such radiation include certain medical treatments and radiation fallout from power plant accidents or nuclear weapons. Having a history of head or neck radiation treatments in childhood is a risk factor for thyroid cancer. In the past, children were sometimes treated with radiation for things we wouldn't use radiation for today, such as acne, fungal infections of the scalp (ringworm), an enlarged thymus gland, or to shrink tonsils or adenoids. Years later, studies linked these treatments to an increased risk for thyroid cancer. **Radiation therapy** in childhood for some cancers such as Hodgkin disease also increases risk. In general, the risk is higher with younger children. Radiation exposure as an adult carries little risk for thyroid cancer.

Several studies have pointed to an increased risk for thyroid cancer in children because of radioactive fallout from nuclear weapons or power plant accidents. For instance, thyroid cancer is several times more common than normal in children living near Chernobyl (former Soviet Union), the site of a 1986 nuclear plant accident that exposed millions of people to **radioactivity.** Adults involved with the cleanup after the accident and those who lived near the plant have also had a higher rate of thyroid cancer. Children with more iodine in their diet appeared to have a lower risk for thyroid cancer. Some radioactive fallout occurred over certain regions of the United States after nuclear weapons testing in western states during the 1950s. This exposure was much, much lower than that found around Chernobyl. At such low exposures, a higher risk of thyroid cancer has not been proved. If you are concerned about possible exposure to radioactive fallout, discuss this issue with your doctor.

Hereditary Conditions

Several inherited conditions have been linked to different types of thyroid cancer.

Medullary Thyroid Cancer

About 1 in 5 cases of MTC can be attributed to an inherited abnormal gene. Familial MTC can occur alone, or it can occur along with other tumors.

The combination of familial MTC and tumors of other **endocrine glands** is called **multiple endocrine neoplasia type 2** (**MEN 2**). There are 2 subtypes, **MEN 2a** and **MEN 2b:**

- In MEN 2a, MTC occurs along with **pheochromocytomas** (tumors in the adrenal glands, which are located on top of the kidneys) and with parathyroid gland tumors.
- In MEN 2b, MTC is associated with pheochromocytomas and **neuromas** (benign growths of nerve tissue found on the tongue and elsewhere). This subtype is much less common than MEN 2a.

In these inherited forms of MTC, the cancers often develop during childhood or early adulthood and can spread early. MTC is most aggressive in the MEN 2b syndrome. If MEN 2a, MEN 2b, or isolated familial MTC runs in your family, then you may be at very high risk for development of MTC. Ask your doctor for information about having regular blood tests to look for problems and whether you should consider genetic testing.

Other Thyroid Cancers

People with certain inherited medical conditions are at higher risk for more common forms of thyroid cancer. Higher rates of the disease occur among people with uncommon genetic conditions such as **Gardner syndrome, Cowden disease,** and **familial adenomatous polyposis (FAP)**.

Papillary and follicular thyroid cancers do seem to run in some families without a known inherited syndrome; these cases may account for about 5% of thyroid cancers. The genetic basis for these cancers is not totally clear.

Prevention and Detection

Do We Know What Causes Thyroid Cancer?

Although scientists have found that thyroid cancer is linked with a number of other conditions (described in the section "What Are the Risk Factors for Thyroid Cancer?" on page 13), the exact cause of most thyroid cancers is not yet known.

Researchers have made great progress in understanding how certain changes in a person's DNA can cause thyroid cells to become cancerous. DNA is the chemical in each of the cells that makes up the **genes**—the instructions for how cells function.

We usually resemble our parents because they are the source of our DNA. However, DNA affects more than how we look. It also can influence our risk for developing certain diseases, including some kinds of cancer.

Some genes contain instructions for controlling when our cells grow and divide. Certain genes that speed up cell division are called **oncogenes.** Others that slow down cell division or cause cells to die at the appropriate time are called **tumor suppressor**

genes. Cancers can be caused by DNA **mutations** (defects) that turn on oncogenes or turn off tumor suppressor genes. People inherit 2 copies of each gene—1 from each parent. People can inherit damaged DNA from 1 or both parents, which accounts for inherited cancers. Most cancers, though, are not inherited. In these cases, a person's DNA is damaged by exposure to something in the environment, like smoke or radiation. Sometimes DNA mutates for no apparent reason.

Papillary Thyroid Cancer

Several DNA mutations have been found to be involved in some forms of papillary thyroid cancer. Many of these cancers have changes in specific parts of the *RET* gene. The altered form of this gene, known as the *PTC* oncogene, is found in about 10% to 30% of papillary thyroid cancers overall and in a larger percentage in children with radiation exposure. Rather than being inherited, these *RET* mutations usually are acquired during a person's lifetime. They are present only in the cancer cells and are not passed on to the patient's children.

Many papillary thyroid cancers (30% to 70%) contain a mutation of the *BRAF* gene. The *BRAF* mutation is less common in thyroid cancers in children and in those believed to arise from exposure to radiation. Cancers with *BRAF* changes tend to grow more aggressively and have a greater likelihood of spreading to other parts of the body. Both

BRAF and *RET/PTC* changes are believed to cause cells to grow and divide. It is extremely rare for papillary cancer to have changes in both the *BRAF* and *RET/PTC* genes. Changes to other genes have also been tied to papillary thyroid cancer, including those in the *NTRK1* gene and the *MET* gene.

Follicular Thyroid Cancer

Acquired changes in the *RAS* oncogene have a role in causing follicular thyroid cancer.

Anaplastic Thyroid Cancer

Anaplastic thyroid cancer tends to have some of the mutations described above, as well as changes in the *p53* tumor suppressor gene.

Medullary Thyroid Cancer

Mutations in people who have MTC involve different parts of the *RET* gene than that seen in papillary carcinoma patients. Nearly all patients with the inherited form of MTC and about 1 of every 5 with the sporadic (noninherited) form of MTC have a mutation in the *RET* gene. Most patients with sporadic MTC have acquired mutations present only in their cancer cells. Those with familial MTC and MEN 2 inherit the *RET* mutation from a parent. These mutations are present in every cell of the patient's body and can be detected by testing the DNA of blood cells. Because every person has 2 *RET* genes but passes only 1 to a child (the child's other *RET* gene comes from the other parent), the odds that a person with familial MTC will pass a mutated gene on to a child are 1 in 2 (or 50%).

Can Thyroid Cancer Be Prevented?

Most people with thyroid cancer have no known risk factors, so it is not possible to prevent most cases of this disease.

Radiation exposure, especially in childhood, is a known risk factor for thyroid cancer. Because of this, doctors no longer use radiation treatment for less serious diseases. In general, it is a good idea to avoid exposing children to any x-rays that aren't necessary.

Genetic blood tests are now available to test for the mutations found in familial MTC. Because of these tests, most of the familial cases of MTC can be prevented or treated early by removing the thyroid gland. Once the disease is discovered in a family, the rest of the family members can be tested for the mutated gene.

If you have a family history of MTC, it is important that you see a doctor who is familiar with the latest advances in **genetic counseling** and **genetic testing** for this disease. Removing the thyroid gland in children who carry the abnormal gene will prevent a cancer that might otherwise be fatal.

Can Thyroid Cancer Be Found Early?

Many cases of thyroid cancer can be found early. In fact, most thyroid cancers are now found much earlier than in the past and can be treated successfully. Most early thyroid cancers are found when patients ask their doctors about lumps or nodules they have noticed. Others are found by health care professionals during routine checkups. Some thyroid cancers may not cause symptoms until after they have reached an advanced stage, but this is rare.

If you have unusual symptoms such as a lump or swelling in your neck, you should make an appointment to see your doctor right away. During a routine physical examination, be sure your doctor does a cancer-related checkup that should include an examination of the thyroid. Some doctors recommend that people examine their own necks twice a year to look for any growths or lumps. Whereas changes in the thyroid can often be detected by blood tests, regular blood tests are not recommended to screen for sporadic (not familial) thyroid cancers.

People with a family history of MTC with or without type 2 multiple endocrine neoplasia (MEN 2) may be at very high risk for development of this cancer. Most doctors recommend genetic testing for these people when they are young to see whether they carry the genetic links to MTC. For people who may be at risk but don't get genetic testing, blood tests are available that can help find MTC at an early stage, when it may still be curable.

Diagnosis and Staging

How Is Thyroid Cancer Diagnosed?

Signs and Symptoms of Thyroid Cancer

Prompt attention to **signs** and **symptoms** is the best approach to early **diagnosis** of most thyroid cancers. Thyroid cancer can cause any of the following local signs or symptoms:

- a lump or swelling in the neck, sometimes growing rapidly
- a pain in the front of the neck, sometimes going up to the ears
- hoarseness or other voice change that does not go away
- trouble swallowing
- breathing problems (feeling as if one were "breathing through a straw")
- a cough that continues and is not due to a cold

If you have any of these signs or symptoms, talk to your doctor right away. Many noncancerous conditions (and some other cancers of the neck area) can cause some of the same symptoms. Thyroid nodules are common and are usually benign.

But the only way to find out for sure is to have a medical evaluation. The sooner you receive a correct diagnosis, the sooner you can start treatment and the more effective your treatment will be.

History and Physical Examination

If you have any signs or symptoms that suggest you might have thyroid cancer, your health care professional will want to take a complete medical history. You will be asked questions about your possible risk factors, symptoms, and any other health problems or concerns. If someone in your family has had thyroid cancer (especially MTC) or adrenal gland tumors called pheochromocytomas, it is important to tell your doctor, as this might indicate you are at higher risk for this disease. A physical examination will give more information about signs of thyroid cancer and other health problems. During the examination, your doctor will pay special attention to the size and firmness of your thyroid and any enlarged lymph nodes in your neck.

Fine Needle Aspiration Biopsy

The actual diagnosis of thyroid cancer is made by a **biopsy,** the process in which cells from a suspicious area are removed and looked at under a microscope. The simplest way to find out whether a thyroid lump or nodule is cancerous is with **fine needle aspiration** of the thyroid nodule. This type of biopsy can usually be done in your doctor's office or clinic. Your doctor will place a thin, hollow needle directly into the nodule to take out cells and a few drops of fluid. The doctor usually repeats this process 2 or 3 times to get samples from several areas of the nodule. The cells can then be viewed under a microscope to see if they look cancerous or benign.

Before the biopsy, local **anesthesia** (numbing medicine) may be injected into the skin over the nodule, but in some cases an **anesthetic** may not be needed. A potential complication of the biopsy is prolonged bleeding, but this complication is rare except in people with bleeding disorders. Be sure to tell your doctor if you have a bleeding disorder.

Fine needle aspiration biopsies are generally done on all thyroid nodules that are large enough to be felt—larger than about 1 cm (about 1/2 inch) across. If a nodule is too small for the doctor to feel, sometimes fine needle aspiration biopsies can be done by using an ultrasound machine to help the doctor find the right place to put the needle.

About 2 in every 10 tests may need to be repeated because the sample ends up not containing enough cells. About 7 of 10 fine needle aspiration biopsies will show that the nodule is benign. Cancer is clearly diagnosed in only 1 of every 20 fine needle aspiration biopsies. Sometimes the test results come back as "suspicious" or "atypical." This outcome happens when the findings of fine needle aspiration biopsy do not clearly show whether the nodule is benign or malignant. In these cases, a more involved biopsy may be needed to get a better sample, particularly if the doctor has reason to think the nodule is cancerous.

Additional procedures may involve using a larger needle for the biopsy, or a surgical "open" biopsy or **lobectomy** (removal of the gland on one side of the windpipe) may be performed. Surgical biopsies are done in an operating room with the patient under general anesthesia (in a deep sleep).

Imaging Tests

Imaging tests may be done for a number of reasons, including to find out whether a suspicious area might be cancerous, to learn how far cancer may have spread, and to help determine whether treatment has been effective.

Chest X-ray

A plain **x-ray** of your chest may be done to see whether cancer has spread to your lungs, especially if you have follicular thyroid cancer.

Ultrasound

Ultrasound, or **sonography,** uses sound waves to create images of your body. For this test, a small, microphone-like instrument called a **transducer** is placed on the skin in front of your thyroid gland. It emits sound waves and picks up the echoes as they bounce off the thyroid gland. The echoes are converted by a computer into a black-and-white image that is displayed on a computer screen. You are not exposed to radiation during this test. This test is helpful in determining whether a thyroid nodule is solid or filled with fluid. It can also be used to check the number and size of thyroid nodules. However, thyroid cancers and most benign nodules can look the same on ultrasound, so this test on its own can't tell whether a nodule is cancerous. For thyroid nodules that are too small to be felt, this test can be used to guide a biopsy needle into the nodule to obtain a sample. Ultrasound can also help determine whether any nearby lymph nodes are enlarged due to spread of the thyroid cancer.

Computed Tomography (CT)

The **CT** or **CAT scan** is an x-ray test that produces detailed cross-sectional images of your body. Instead of taking one picture, like a regular x-ray, a CT scanner takes many pictures as it rotates around you while you lie on a table. A computer then combines these pictures into images of "slices" of the part of your body being studied. Unlike a regular x-ray, a CT scan creates images of the soft tissues in the body.

After the first set of pictures is taken, you may be asked to drink a contrast solution or receive an intravenous (IV) line through which a contrast dye is injected. This helps better outline the structures in your body. A second set of pictures is then taken. The contrast may cause some flushing (a feeling of warmth, especially in the face). Some people are allergic to the contrast dye and get hives. A more serious reaction like trouble breathing or low blood pressure can occur, but this is rare. Be sure to tell the doctor if you have ever had a reaction to any contrast material used for x-rays.

CT scans take longer than regular x-rays. You need to lie still on a table while they are being done. During the test, the table moves in and out of the scanner, a ring-shaped machine that completely surrounds the table. You might feel a bit confined by the machine in which you have to lie while the pictures are being taken. The CT scan can help determine the location and size of thyroid cancers and whether they have spread to nearby areas, although ultrasound is usually the test of choice. A CT scan can also be used to look for spread in distant organs such as the lungs. In some cases, a CT scan can be used to guide a biopsy needle precisely into a suspected area of metastasis. For a **CT–guided needle biopsy,** the patient remains on the CT scanning table while a radiologist advances a biopsy needle toward the location of the mass. CT scans are repeated until the doctor can see that the needle is within the mass. A biopsy sample is then removed and examined under a microscope.

Magnetic Resonance Imaging (MRI)

Like CT scans, **MRI** scans can be used to look for cancer in the thyroid or cancer spread to nearby or distant parts of the body, although ultrasound is usually the first choice. MRI can provide very detailed images of soft tissues such as the thyroid gland. MRI scans are also particularly helpful in looking at the brain and spinal cord. MRI scans use radio waves and strong magnets instead of x-rays. The energy from the radio waves is absorbed and then released in a pattern formed by the type of body tissue and by certain diseases. A computer translates the pattern into a very detailed image of parts of the body. A contrast material called

gadolinium is often injected into a vein before the scan to better show details.

MRI scanning causes more discomfort than CT scanning. First, the MRI takes longer to perform—often up to an hour. Second, you have to lie inside a narrow tube, which is confining and can upset people with claustrophobia (a fear of enclosed spaces). Newer, "open" MRI machines may minimize this effect. MRI machines also make buzzing and clicking noises that some people find disturbing. Some centers provide headphones with music to block out this noise.

Nuclear Medicine Scans

Nuclear medicine (**radionuclide**) **scanning** involves inserting small amounts of radioactive substances into the body; then, special cameras are used to detect where the substances go. These tests can help locate cells in your body that are not behaving normally, although these scans don't provide very detailed images.

Radioiodine Scan

For this test, a small amount of **radioactive iodine** is swallowed (usually as a pill) or injected into a vein. The iodine is absorbed by the thyroid gland (or thyroid cells anywhere in the body) over time, and several hours later a special camera is used to see where the radioactivity has gone. For a "thyroid scan," the camera is placed in front of your neck to measure the amount of radiation in the gland. Abnormal areas of the thyroid that contain less radioactivity than the surrounding tissue are called **cold nodules,** and areas that take up more radiation are called **hot nodules.** Hot nodules are not usually cancerous, but cold nodules can be benign or cancerous. Because both benign and cancerous nodules can appear cold, this test alone is not sufficient to diagnose thyroid cancer.

Radioiodine scans are frequently used in the care and management of patients with differentiated thyroid cancer (papillary and follicular [including Hürthle cell]). Because MTC cells do not take up iodine, radioiodine scans are not used for this cancer. If a biopsy has been performed and shows that thyroid cancer is present, whole-body radioiodine scans are very useful in follow-up, to show potential spread of differentiated thyroid cancers throughout the body. Scans after surgery can also help determine how far a thyroid cancer has spread, if at all.

If the entire thyroid gland has been removed because of cancer, radioiodine scans may be done frequently. The scan is more sensitive under these circumstances because more of the radioactive iodine is picked up by thyroid cancer cells that have spread elsewhere in the body.

Radioiodine scans work best if patients have high blood levels of thyroid-stimulating hormone (**TSH,** or **thyrotropin**). You can increase your level of TSH by stopping your thyroid hormone pills for a few days to a few weeks before the test. Temporarily stopping this medication lowers your thyroid hormone levels and causes the pituitary gland to release more TSH, which in turn stimulates the cancer cells to take up the radioactive iodine. Although this intentional hypothyroidism is temporary, it can cause symptoms like tiredness, depression, weight gain, sleepiness, constipation, muscle aches, and reduced concentration. An injectable form of thyrotropin is now available that can increase patients' TSH levels before radio-iodine scanning, so withholding thyroid hormone for a long period may not be necessary. Because iodine already in the body can interfere with this test, people are usually told not to ingest foods or medicines that contain iodine in the days before the scan.

Positron Emission Tomography (PET) Scan

PET scans involve injecting glucose (a form of sugar) that contains a radioactive atom into the blood. Because cancer cells in the body are growing rapidly, they absorb large amounts of the radioactive sugar. A special camera can then be used to create a picture of areas of radioactivity in the body. This test can be very useful if you have a type of thyroid cancer that doesn't take up radioac-tive iodine. In this situation, the PET scan may be able to show whether the cancer has spread. Some newer machines are able to perform both a PET and CT scan at the same time (PET/CT scan), allowing the doctor to see areas that "light up" on the PET scan in more detail.

Octreotide Scan

Sometimes an **octreotide scan,** which uses a radioactively labeled hormone, may be done to look for the spread of MTC. These cancers don't take up iodine, so radioiodine scans cannot be used for them.

Blood Tests

No blood test can tell whether a thyroid nodule is cancerous. However, tests of blood levels of thyroid-stimulating hormone (TSH) may be used to check the overall activity of your thyroid gland. Levels of thyroid hormones (T3 and T4) may also be measured to get a sense of thyroid gland function.

Thyroglobulin is a protein made by the thyroid gland. Its measurement cannot be used to diagnose thyroid cancer. But after most of the thyroid has been removed by surgery and the remaining normal cells destroyed by radioactive iodine, levels of thyroglobulin in the blood should be very low. If they are not low, this might mean that thyroid cancer is still present. If the level rises, it is a sign that the cancer may be coming back.

If MTC is suspected or if you have a family history of the disease, blood tests for calcitonin levels can help tell whether MTC is present. This test is also useful after treatment of MTC to look for possible **recurrence.** Because calcitonin can affect blood calcium levels, these levels may be checked as well. People with MTC often have high blood levels of a protein called carcinoembryonic antigen (CEA). Tests for CEA can sometimes help tell whether cancer is present. You may have other blood tests as well. For example, if you are scheduled for surgery, tests will be done to check your blood cell counts, to look for bleeding disorders, and to check the function of your liver and kidneys.

How Is Thyroid Cancer Staged?

Staging is the process of finding out whether a cancer has spread and, if so, how far. The stage of a cancer is one of the most important factors in choosing treatment options and predicting your chance for cure and long-term survival. Staging is based on the results of the physical examination, biopsy, and imaging tests (ultrasound, CT scan, MRI, chest x-ray, and/or nuclear medicine scans), which are described in the section, "How Is Thyroid Cancer Diagnosed?" on page 23.

The TNM Staging System

A staging system is a standard way for the **cancer care team** to summarize the size of a tumor and how far the cancer has spread. Ask your doctor to explain thyroid cancer staging in a way that you understand so that you can take a more active role in making informed decisions about your treatment.

The most common system used to describe the stages of cancer is the **American Joint Committee on Cancer (AJCC) TNM system.** The **TNM system** describes 3 key pieces of information:

- **T** indicates the size of the main (primary) **tumor** and whether it has grown into nearby areas.
- **N** describes the extent of spread to nearby (regional) lymph **nodes.** Lymph nodes are

small, bean-shaped collections of immune system cells that are important in fighting infections.

- **M** indicates whether the cancer has spread (**metastasized**) to other organs of the body. (The most common site of spread is to the lungs. The next most common sites are the liver and bones.)

Numbers or letters appear after T, N, and M to provide more details about each of these factors. The numbers 0 through 4 indicate increasing severity. The letter X means "cannot be assessed because the information is not available."

T categories for thyroid cancer:

TX: Primary tumor cannot be assessed

T0: No evidence of primary tumor

T1: The tumor is 2 cm (slightly less than an inch) across or smaller

T2: Tumor is between 2 cm and 4 cm (slightly less than 2 inches) across

T3: Tumor is larger than 4 cm or has begun to grow into nearby tissues outside the thyroid

T4a: Tumor may be any size and has spread extensively beyond the thyroid gland into nearby tissues of the neck

T4b: Tumor has grown either back toward the spine or into nearby large blood vessels

For anaplastic thyroid cancers:

T4a: Tumor is still within the thyroid and may be resectable (removable by surgery)

T4b: Tumor has grown outside of the thyroid and is not resectable

N categories for thyroid cancer:

NX: Regional (nearby) lymph nodes cannot be assessed

N0: No spread to nearby lymph nodes

N1: Spread to nearby lymph nodes

N1a: Spread to lymph nodes around the thyroid in the neck (cervical)

N1b: Spread to lymph nodes in the sides of the neck (lateral cervical) or the upper chest (upper mediastinal)

M categories for thyroid cancer:

MX: Presence of distant metastasis (spread) cannot be assessed

M0: No distant metastasis

M1: Distant metastasis is present, involving distant lymph nodes, internal organs, bones, etc.

Stage Grouping

To make this information clearer, TNM descriptions can be grouped together into stage I through stage IV. Unlike most other cancers, thyroid cancers are grouped into stages in a way that considers both the subtype of cancer and the patient's age.

Stage Grouping for Papillary or Follicular Thyroid Carcinoma (Differentiated Thyroid Cancer)

Younger people are less likely to die of differentiated (papillary or follicular) thyroid cancer.

The TNM stage groupings for these cancers take this fact into account. So, for example, all people younger than age 45 with papillary thyroid cancer are *stage I* if they have no distant spread and *stage II* if they have distant metastases beyond the neck or upper mediastinal lymph nodes.

Patients younger than age 45:

Stage I (any T, any N, M0): The tumor can be any size and may or may not have spread to nearby lymph nodes. It has not spread to distant sites.

Stage II (any T, any N, M1): The tumor can be any size and may or may not have spread to nearby lymph nodes. It has spread to distant sites.

Patients 45 years of age and older:

Stage I (T1, N0, M0): The tumor is less than 2 cm across and has not spread to nearby lymph nodes or distant sites.

Stage II (T2, N0, M0): The tumor is 2 cm to 4 cm across and has not spread to nearby lymph nodes or distant sites.

Stage III (T3, N0, M0 or T1-3, N1a, M0): One of the following applies:

- The tumor is larger than 4 cm or has grown slightly outside the thyroid, but it has not spread to nearby lymph nodes or distant sites.
- The tumor is any size and has spread to lymph nodes around the thyroid in the

neck (cervical nodes) but not to distant sites.

Stage IVA (T4a, N0-1a, M0 or T1-4, N1b, M0): One of the following applies:

- The tumor is any size and has grown beyond the thyroid gland to invade nearby tissues of the neck. It may or may not have spread to lymph nodes around the thyroid in the neck (cervical nodes). It has not spread to distant sites.
- The tumor is any size and may have grown outside of the thyroid gland. It has spread to lymph nodes in the side of the neck (lateral cervical nodes) or upper chest (upper mediastinal nodes) but not to distant sites.

Stage IVB (T4b, any N, M0): The tumor is any size and has grown either back to the spine or into nearby large blood vessels. It may or may not have spread to nearby lymph nodes, but it has not spread to distant sites.

Stage IVC (any T, any N, M1): The tumor is any size and may or may not have grown outside the thyroid. It may or may not have spread to nearby lymph nodes. It has spread to distant sites.

Stage Grouping for MTC

Stage grouping for MTC in people of any age is the same as for papillary or follicular carcinoma in people older than age 45.

Stage Grouping for Anaplastic/Undifferentiated Thyroid Carcinoma

All anaplastic thyroid cancers are considered stage IV, reflecting the poor prognosis of this type of cancer.

Stage IVA (T4a, any N, M0): Tumor is still within the thyroid and may be resectable (removable by surgery). It may or may not have spread to nearby lymph nodes, but it has not spread to distant sites.

Stage IVB (T4b, any N, M0): Tumor has grown outside of the thyroid and is not resectable. It may or may not have spread to nearby lymph nodes, but it has not spread to distant sites.

Stage IVC (any T, any N, M1): The tumor is any size and may or may not have grown outside of the thyroid. It may or may not have spread to nearby lymph nodes. It has spread to distant sites.

Recurrent (Relapsed) Cancer

This is not an actual stage in the TNM system. Recurrent (relapsed) disease means that the cancer has come back (recurred) after treatment. Thyroid cancer usually returns in the neck, but it may reappear in another part of the body (for example, lymph nodes, lungs, bones). Doctors may assign a new stage based on how far the cancer has spread, but this is not usually as formal a process as the original staging. The presence of recurrent disease does not change the original, formal staging.

If you have any questions about the stage of your cancer or how it affects your treatment, do not hesitate to ask your doctor.

Thyroid Cancer Survival, by Type and Stage

The following survival statistics come from the *AJCC Cancer Staging Manual* (6th ed). There are some important points to note about these numbers:

- The **5-year survival rate** refers to the percentage of patients who live *at least 5 years* after being diagnosed. Many of these patients live much longer than 5 years after diagnosis. **Five-year relative survival rates** (such as the rates shown below) don't include patients who die of other causes. They are considered to be a more accurate way to describe the outlook for patients with a particular type and stage of cancer.

- These numbers were derived from patients treated between 1985 and 1991. While these numbers are among the most current we have available, they represent people who were first diagnosed and treated at least 15 to 20 years ago. Improvement in treatment since then means that the outlook for people now being diagnosed with these cancers is likely to be better.

- While survival statistics can sometimes be useful as a general guide, they may not accurately represent any one person's prognosis. A number of other factors, including other tumor characteristics and a person's age and general health, can also affect outlook. Your doctor is likely to know whether these numbers apply to you, as he or she is familiar with your particular situation.

Five-Year Relative Survival Rates for Anaplastic Thyroid Cancer

The 5-year relative survival rate for anaplastic (undifferentiated) carcinomas, all of which are considered stage IV, is around 9%.

Five-Year Relative Survival Rates

Papillary Thyroid Cancer

Stage	5-Year Relative Survival Rate (%)
I	100
II	100
III	96
IV	45

Follicular Thyroid Cancer

Stage	5-Year Relative Survival Rate (%)
I	100
II	100
III	79
IV	47

MTC

Stage	5-Year Relative Survival Rate (%)
I	100
II	97
III	78
IV	24

Note: All patients with stage III or IV disease are, by definition, over 45 years old.

Treatment

How Is Thyroid Cancer Treated?

The methods of treatment for thyroid cancer include surgery, radioiodine treatment, thyroid hormone therapy, external beam radiation therapy, and chemotherapy. The best approach often uses 2 or more of these methods; most patients are cured of their thyroid cancer in this way. If a cure is not possible, the goal may be to remove or destroy as much of the cancer as possible and to prevent the tumor from growing, spreading, or returning for as long as possible. Sometimes treatment is aimed at **palliation** (relieving symptoms, such as pain or problems with breathing and swallowing). Read more about **palliative treatment** on pages 88–89.

Making Treatment Decisions

After thyroid cancer is found, your doctor will discuss treatment options with you. It is important to take the time to consider each of them. In choosing a treatment plan, factors to consider include the type and stage of the cancer and your general health. If you have any concerns about your treatment plan, it is a good idea to get a second opinion. In fact, many doctors encourage this step. Some insurance companies even require a second opinion before they will agree to pay for certain treatments. A second opinion can provide more information and help you feel confident about the treatment plan you choose.

The next part of this section describes the various treatments used for thyroid cancers, followed by a description of the most common approaches based on the type and stage of the cancer. The last part of the section describes members of the cancer care team who might be involved in your care.

Surgery

Surgery is the main treatment for thyroid cancer and is used in nearly every case, except perhaps for some anaplastic thyroid cancers. If the results of fine needle aspiration biopsies indicate thyroid cancer, surgery to remove the tumor and all or part of the remaining thyroid gland is usually recommended.

Different types of surgery for thyroid cancer are described below.

Lobectomy

Lobectomy is sometimes used for differentiated thyroid cancers that are small and show no signs of having spread beyond the thyroid gland. The lobe containing the cancer is removed, usually along with the **isthmus** (the small piece of the gland that acts as a "bridge" between the left and right lobes; see diagram on page 3). Because this surgery does not remove the unaffected lobe and the thyroid **cartilage,** lifelong use of thyroid hormone supplements may not be needed afterward. However, having some of the thyroid gland remaining can interfere with some tests to look for cancer recurrence after treatment, such as radio-iodine scans.

Thyroidectomy

Thyroidectomy removes all (total **thyroidectomy**), nearly all (near-total thyroidectomy), or most (subtotal thyroidectomy) of the thyroid gland. It is the most common surgery for thyroid cancer. It is often used even for differentiated thyroid cancers because papillary thyroid cancer tends to be present in more than one part of the thyroid gland and because follicular cancer is more aggressive.

Lymph Node Removal

When cancer has spread outside the thyroid gland, surgery is always used to remove, as much as possible, any cancer that has invaded the neck, including cancer that has spread to lymph nodes. This is especially true for treatment of MTC and for anaplastic cancer (when surgery is an option).

For papillary or follicular cancer in which only 1 or 2 enlarged lymph nodes are thought to contain cancer, these enlarged nodes may be removed and any small deposits of cancer cells that are left are treated with radioactive iodine (see "Radioactive Iodine Therapy" on page 45). More often, several lymph nodes near the thyroid are removed in an operation called a **central compartment neck dissection.** Removal of more lymph nodes, including those on the side of the neck, is called a **modified radical neck dissection.**

Sentinel lymph node biopsy: Another technique for looking at possible spread to lymph nodes is called a **sentinel lymph node biopsy.** In this procedure, a radioactive tracer and blue dye are injected into the tumor. The dye and radioactive material travel to the lymph nodes where the cancer would likely spread. The surgeon then removes the sentinel node—the first lymph node into which a tumor drains and usually the one most likely to contain cancer cells. If the sentinel node is cancer-free, no other lymph nodes are removed. While this technique is commonly used for some other cancers, the benefit of sentinel lymph node biopsy for thyroid cancer is still unclear.

Risks and Side Effects of Surgery

Patients who have thyroid surgery are often ready to leave the hospital within a few days after the operation. Potential complications of thyroid surgery include the following:

- temporary or permanent hoarseness or loss of voice (this can happen if the larynx [voice box] or windpipe is irritated by the breathing tube that was used during surgery or if the nerves to the larynx are damaged during surgery)
- damage to the parathyroid glands (small glands near the thyroid that help regulate blood calcium levels), which can lead to low blood calcium levels, causing muscle spasms and numbness and tingling sensations in the neck

- excessive bleeding or formation of a major blood clot (hematoma) in the neck
- wound infection
- pain that is usually mild and not long lasting

Most doctors recommend that a surgeon experienced in treating thyroid cancer perform the surgery. Complications are less likely to happen when you have an experienced thyroid surgeon, especially one with specialized training. If most or all of your thyroid gland is removed, you will need to take daily thyroid hormone replacement pills. All patients who have had near-total or total thyroidectomy will need this supplement.

Radioactive Iodine (Radioiodine) Therapy

Your thyroid gland absorbs nearly all of the iodine in your blood. When a form of radioactive iodine known as **RAI I-131** is taken into the body, it can destroy the thyroid gland and any other thyroid cells (including cancer cells) that take up iodine without affecting the rest of your body. (The radiation dose used here is much stronger than the one used in radioiodine scans, described in "How Is Thyroid Cancer Diagnosed?" on pages 29–31.) The radioactive iodine is usually given as a capsule or liquid. This treatment can be used to ablate (destroy) any thyroid tissue not removed by surgery or to treat thyroid cancer that has spread to lymph nodes and other parts of the body.

Radioactive iodine therapy has been shown to improve the survival rate of patients with papillary or follicular thyroid cancer (differentiated thyroid cancer) that has spread to the neck or other body parts, and this treatment is now standard practice in such cases. But the benefits of radioactive iodine therapy are less clear for patients with small cancers of the thyroid gland that have not spread. Radioactive iodine therapy is not used to treat anaplastic (undifferentiated) and MTCs because these types of cancer do not take up iodine.

For radioactive iodine therapy to be most effective, patients must have high levels of thyroid-stimulating hormone (TSH, or thyrotropin) in the blood. This substance stimulates thyroid tissue (and cancer cells) to take up radioactive iodine. After surgery, TSH levels can be raised by stopping thyroid hormone pills for several weeks. Stopping this medication causes very low thyroid hormone levels (a condition known as hypothyroidism), which in turn causes the pituitary gland to release more TSH. Although this intentional hypothyroidism is temporary, it can cause symptoms like tiredness, depression, weight gain, sleepiness, constipation, muscle aches, and reduced concentration. An injectable form of thyrotropin that can increase the TSH levels is now available. It is sometimes used before thyroid scans, but it is not clear whether it is as effective as stopping thyroid hormones for radioactive iodine therapy.

Risks and Side Effects of Radioactive Iodine Therapy

Depending on the dose of radioactive iodine used and where you are being treated, you may need to be in the hospital for up to a few days after treatment, staying in a special isolation room to prevent others from being exposed to radiation. Some people may not need to be hospitalized. You may be allowed to go home after treatment. If this is the case, you will be given instructions on how to protect others from radiation exposure.

Short-term **side effects** of radioactive iodine treatment may include the following:

- neck tenderness
- nausea and upset stomach
- swelling and tenderness of the salivary glands
- dry mouth
- taste changes
- pain (this is rare)

Chewing gum or sucking on hard candy may help with salivary gland problems. Radioiodine treatment also reduces tear formation in some people, leading to dry eyes.

Men who receive large total doses because of many treatments with radioactive iodine may have lower sperm counts or, rarely, may become infertile. Radioactive iodine may also affect a woman's ovaries, and some women may have irregular periods for up to a year after treatment. Many doctors recommend that women avoid becoming pregnant for 6 months to a year after treatment.

Both men and women who have had radioactive iodine therapy may have a slightly increased risk for development of leukemia in the future. Doctors disagree on exactly how much this risk is increased, but most of the largest studies have found that this complication is extremely rare. Some research even suggests the risk for leukemia may not be significantly increased.

Thyroid Hormone Therapy

After a thyroidectomy, the body is no longer able to make the thyroid hormone it needs, so patients must daily take thyroid hormone pills to replace the loss of the natural hormone. Replacement is lifelong.

Thyroid therapy can serve 2 purposes:

- to help maintain the body's normal metabolism (by replacing missing thyroid hormone)
- to help stop cancer cells from growing (by lowering TSH levels)

Thyroid hormone may also help prevent some thyroid cancers from returning. Normal thyroid function is regulated by the pituitary gland. The pituitary gland makes TSH, which causes the thyroid gland to make thyroid hormone for the body. TSH also promotes growth of the thyroid gland and thyroid cancer cells. The level of TSH, in turn, is regulated by how much thyroid hormone is in the blood. If the level of thyroid hormone is low, the pituitary gland makes more TSH. If the level of thyroid hormone is high, not as much TSH is needed, so the pituitary gland makes less of it. Doctors have learned that by giving higher than normal doses of thyroid hormone, TSH levels can be kept very low. This effect may slow the growth of cancer cells and lower the chance of having some cancers (especially high-risk cancers) come back.

Possible Side Effects of Thyroid Hormone Therapy

Even though these higher than normal levels of thyroid hormone seem to have few side effects, some doctors have expressed concerns about long-term issues, such as possible effects on the bones and heart. Because of this concern, high doses of thyroid hormone may be reserved for people with differentiated thyroid cancers who are at high risk of recurrence.

External Beam Radiation Therapy

External beam radiation therapy uses high-energy rays (or particles) to destroy cancer cells or slow their rate of growth. A carefully focused beam of radiation is delivered from a machine outside the body. Generally, this type of radiation treatment is not used for cancers that take up iodine (that is, most differentiated thyroid cancers), which can be more effectively treated with radioiodine therapy. External beam radiation therapy is more often used as part of the treatment for MTC and anaplastic thyroid cancer.

When a cancer that does not take up iodine has spread beyond the **thyroid capsule,** external radiation treatment may help treat the cancer or reduce the chance of the disease coming back in the neck after surgery. If a cancer does not respond to radioiodine therapy, external radiation therapy may be used to treat local neck recurrence or distant metastases that are causing pain or other symptoms. External beam radiation therapy usually involves treatments 5 days a week for about 6 weeks. The treatment itself is painless and much like getting a regular x-ray. Each treatment lasts only a few minutes, although the setup time—getting you into place for treatment—usually takes longer.

Possible Side Effects of External Beam Radiation Therapy

The main drawback of this treatment is that the radiation can destroy nearby healthy tissue along with the cancer cells. Some patients get skin changes similar to sunburn, but this result slowly fades away. Trouble swallowing, hoarseness, and fatigue are also potential side effects of external beam radiation therapy. To reduce the risk of side effects, doctors carefully figure out the exact dose needed and aim the beam as accurately as they can to hit the target.

For more information about radiation therapy, see the American Cancer Society document *Understanding Radiation Therapy: A Guide for Patients and Families*, available on the Web at **www.cancer.org** or by calling **800-ACS-2345.**

Chemotherapy

Chemotherapy is the use of anticancer drugs that are injected into a vein or a muscle or taken by mouth. Chemotherapy is **systemic therapy,** which means that the drug enters the bloodstream and circulates throughout the body to reach and destroy the cancer cells. Only some types of thyroid cancer respond to chemotherapy. It is combined with external beam radiation therapy for anaplastic thyroid cancer and is sometimes used for other advanced cancers that are no longer responding to other treatments.

Possible Side Effects of Chemotherapy

Chemotherapy drugs work by attacking cells that are dividing quickly, which is why they work against cancer cells. But other cells in the body, such as those in the hair follicles, bone marrow, and the lining of the mouth and intestines also divide quickly. These cells are also likely to be affected by chemotherapy, which can cause side effects.

The side effects of chemotherapy depend on the type and dose of drugs given and the length of time they are taken. These side effects can include the following:

- hair loss
- mouth sores
- loss of appetite
- nausea and vomiting
- increased chance of infections (due to low white blood cell counts)
- easy bruising or bleeding (due to low blood platelet counts)
- fatigue (due to low red blood cell counts)

These side effects are usually short-term and go away after treatment is finished. There are often ways to lessen these side effects. For example, drugs can be given to help prevent or reduce nausea and vomiting.

For more information about chemotherapy, see the American Cancer Society document *Understanding Chemotherapy: A Guide for Patients and Families* available on the Web at **www.cancer.org** or by calling **800-ACS-2345.**

Clinical Trials

If you have been told you have thyroid cancer, you have a lot of decisions to make. One of the most important decisions you will make is deciding which treatment is best for you. You may have heard about clinical trials being done for your type of cancer. Or maybe someone on your health care team has mentioned a clinical trial to you. Clinical trials are one way to get state-of-the art cancer care. Still, they are not right for everyone.

Here we will give you a brief overview of clinical trials. Talking to your health care team, your family, and your friends can help you make the best treatment choices.

Clinical trials are carefully controlled research studies that are done with patients. These studies test whether a new treatment is safe and how well it works in patients, or they may test new ways to diagnose or prevent a disease. Clinical trials have led to many advances in cancer prevention, diagnosis, and treatment.

Clinical trials are done to get a closer look at promising new treatments or procedures in patients. A clinical trial is undertaken only when there is good reason to believe that the treatment, test, or procedure being studied may be better than the one already being used. Treatments used in clinical trials are often found to have real benefits and may go on to become tomorrow's standard treatment.

Clinical trials can focus on many things:

- new uses of drugs that are already approved by the U.S. Food and Drug Administration (FDA)
- new drugs that have not yet been approved by the FDA
- nondrug treatments (such as radiation therapy)
- medical procedures (such as types of surgery)
- herbs and vitamins
- tools to improve the ways medicines or diagnostic tests are used
- medicines or procedures to relieve symptoms or improve comfort
- combinations of treatments and procedures

Researchers conduct studies of new treatments to try to answer the following questions:

- Is the treatment helpful?
- What's the best way to give it?
- Does it work better than other treatments already available?
- What side effects does the treatment cause?
- Are there more or fewer side effects than those associated with the standard treatment used now?
- Do the benefits outweigh the side effects?
- In which patients is the treatment most likely to be helpful?

There are 4 phases of clinical trials, which are numbered I, II, III, and IV. We will use the example of testing a new cancer treatment drug to look at what each phase is like.

Phase I Clinical Trials

The purpose of a phase I study is to find the safest way to give a new treatment to patients. The cancer care team closely watches patients for any harmful side effects.

For phase I studies, the drug has already been tested in laboratory and animal studies, but the side effects in patients are not fully known. Doctors start by giving very low doses of the drug to the first patients and increase the doses for later groups of patients until side effects appear or the desired effect is seen. Doctors are hoping to help the study patients, but the main purpose of a phase I trial is to test the safety of the drug.

Phase I clinical trials are often done in small groups of people with different cancers that have not responded to standard treatment, or that keep coming back (recurring) after treatment. If a drug is found to be reasonably safe in phase I studies, it can be tested in a phase II clinical trial.

Phase II Clinical Trials

These studies are designed to see whether the drug is effective. Patients are given the most appropriate (safest) dose as determined from phase I studies. They are closely watched for an effect on the cancer. The cancer care team also looks for side effects. Phase II trials are often done in larger groups of patients with a specific cancer type that has not responded to standard treatment. If a drug is found to be effective in phase II studies, it can be tested in a phase III clinical trial.

Phase III Clinical Trials

Phase III studies involve large numbers of patients—most often those patients who have just received a diagnosis for a specific type of cancer. Phase III clinical trials may enroll thousands of patients. Often, these studies are randomized, which means that patients are randomly put in 1 of 2 (or more) groups. One group (called the **control group**) gets the standard, most accepted treatment. The other group(s) gets the new treatment(s) being studied. All patients in phase III studies are closely watched. The study will be stopped early if many patients have side effects from the new treatment that are too severe or if one group has much better results than the others. Phase III clinical trials are needed before the FDA will approve a treatment for use by the general public.

Phase IV Clinical Trials

Once a drug has been approved by the FDA and is available for all patients, it is still studied in other clinical trials (sometimes referred to as phase IV studies). This way, more can be learned about short-term and long-term side effects and safety as the drug is used in larger numbers of patients with many types of diseases. Doctors can also learn more about how well the drug works and whether it might be helpful when used in other ways (such as in combination with other treatments).

What It Is Like to Be in a Clinical Trial

If you participate in a clinical trial, you will have a team of cancer care experts taking care of you and watching your progress very carefully. Depending on the phase of the clinical trial, you may receive more attention (such as having more doctor visits and laboratory tests) than you would if you were treated outside of a clinical trial. Clinical trials are designed to pay close attention to you. However, there are some risks. No one involved in the study knows in advance whether the treatment will work or exactly what side effects will occur. That outcome is what the study is designed to find out. While most side effects go away in time, some may be long-lasting or even life-threatening. Keep in mind, though, that even standard treatments have side effects.

Deciding to Enter a Clinical Trial

If you would like to take part in a clinical trial, you should begin by asking your doctor if your clinic or hospital conducts clinical trials. There are requirements you must meet to take part in any clinical trial. But whether or not you enter (enroll in) a clinical trial is completely up to you. The doctors and nurses conducting the study will explain the study to you in detail. They will go over the possible risks and benefits and give you a form (**informed consent**) to read and sign. The form says that you understand the clinical trial and want to take part in it. Even after you read and sign the form and after the clinical trial begins, you are free to leave the study at any time, for any reason. Taking part in a clinical trial does not keep you from getting any other medical care you may need.

To find out more about clinical trials, talk to your cancer care team. Here are some questions you might ask:

- Is there a clinical trial that I should take part in?
- What is the purpose of the study?
- How might this study be of benefit to me?
- What is likely to happen in my case with, or without, this new treatment?
- What kinds of tests and treatments does the study involve?
- What does this treatment do? Has it been used before?
- Will I know which treatment I receive?
- What are my other choices and their pros and cons?
- How could the study affect my daily life?
- What side effects can I expect from the study? Can the side effects be controlled?
- Will I have to stay in the hospital? If so, how often and for how long?
- Will the study cost me anything? Will any of the treatment be free?
- If I am harmed as a result of the research, what treatment would I be entitled to?
- What type of long-term follow-up care is part of the study?
- Has the treatment been used to treat other types of cancer?

How Can I Find Out More About Clinical Trials that Might Be Right for Me?

The American Cancer Society offers a clinical trials matching service for use by patients, their family, or friends. You can reach this service at **800-303-5691** or on our Web site at **http://clinicaltrials.cancer.org**.

Based on the information you give about your cancer type, stage, and previous treatments, this service can put together a list of clinical trials that match your medical needs. The service will also ask where you live and whether you are willing to travel so that it can look for a treatment center near you. You can also get a list of current clinical trials by calling the National Cancer Institute's Cancer Information Service toll-free at **800-4-CANCER** (**800-422-6237**) or by visiting the NCI clinical trials Web site at **www.cancer.gov/clinicaltrials**.

For more information on clinical trials, see the American Cancer Society document *Clinical Trials: What You Need to Know,* available on the Web at **www.cancer.org** or by calling **800-ACS-2345**.

Complementary and Alternative Treatments

When you have cancer, you are likely to hear about ways to treat your cancer or relieve symptoms that are different from mainstream (**standard**) **medical treatment.** These treatments can include vitamins, herbs, and special diets, or acupuncture and massage—among many others. You may have a lot of questions about these treatments. Talk to your doctor about any treatment you are considering. Here are some questions to ask:

- How do I know if the treatment is safe?
- How do I know if it works?
- Should I try one or more of these treatments?
- Will these treatments cause a problem with my standard medical treatment?
- What is the difference between complementary and alternative treatments?
- Where can I find out more about these treatments?

The Terms Can Be Confusing

Not everyone uses these terms the same way, so it can be confusing. The American Cancer Society uses **complementary medicine** to refer to medicines or treatments that are used along with your regular medical care. **Alternative medicine** is a treatment used instead of standard medical treatment.

Complementary Treatments

Complementary treatment methods, for the most part, are not presented as cures for cancer. Most often they are used to help you feel better. Some methods that can be used in a complementary way are meditation to reduce stress, acupuncture to relieve pain, or peppermint tea to relieve nausea. There are many others. Some of these methods are known to help and could add to your comfort and well-being, while others have not been tested. Some have been proven not to be helpful. A few have even been found harmful. There are many complementary methods that you can safely use right along with your medical treatment to help relieve symptoms or side effects, to ease pain, and to help you enjoy life more. For example, some people find methods such as aromatherapy, massage therapy, meditation, or yoga to be useful.

Alternative Treatments

Alternative treatments are those methods that are used instead of standard medical care. These treatments have not been proven to be safe and effective in clinical trials. Some of these treatments may even be dangerous or have life-threatening side effects. The biggest danger in most cases is that you may lose the chance to benefit from standard treatment. Delays or interruptions in your standard medical treatment may give the cancer more time to grow.

Deciding What to Do

It is easy to see why people with cancer may consider alternative treatments. You want to do all you can to fight the cancer. Sometimes mainstream treatments such as chemotherapy can be hard to take, or they may no longer be working. Sometimes people suggest that their treatment can cure your cancer without having serious side effects, and it's normal to want to believe them. But the truth is that most nonstandard treatments have not been tested and proven to be effective for treating cancer.

As you consider your options, here are 3 important steps you can take:

- Talk to your doctor or nurse about any treatment you are thinking about using.
- Check the list of "red flags," below.
- Contact the American Cancer Society at **800-ACS-2345** to learn more about complementary and alternative treatments in general and to learn more about the specific treatments you are considering.

Red Flags

You can use the questions below to spot treatments or methods to avoid. A "yes" answer to any one of these questions should raise a red flag.

- Does the treatment promise a cure?
- Are you told not to use standard medical treatment?
- Is the treatment or drug a "secret" that only certain people can give?
- Does the treatment require you to travel to another country?
- Do the promoters attack the medical or scientific community?

The Decision Is Yours

Decisions about how to treat or manage your cancer are always yours to make. If you are thinking about using a complementary or alternative method, be sure to learn about it and talk with your doctor about it. With reliable information and the support of your health care team, you may be able to safely use methods that can help you while avoiding those that could be harmful.

Treatment of Thyroid Cancer by Stage

The type of treatment your doctor will recommend depends on the type and stage of the cancer and on your overall health. This section summarizes options usually considered for each type and stage of thyroid cancer.

Papillary Carcinoma and Papillary Carcinoma Variants

Stage I: Lobectomy (removal of only the affected side of the thyroid gland) may be an option if the patient is fairly young, the tumor is small (less than about 1 cm across), and there is no sign of cancer in the lymph nodes or the other thyroid lobe. Thyroidectomy is also an option to treat these cancers. Radioiodine treatment is sometimes used after thyroidectomy, but the cure rate with surgery alone is excellent. In the unlikely event of recurrence, radioiodine treatment can still be offered.

If the patient is younger than age 15 or older than 45, or if the tumor is larger than 1 cm, is growing outside the covering capsule of the thyroid gland, or there is obvious spread to lymph nodes, doctors prefer thyroidectomy, including the removal and microscopic examination of the lymph nodes. Radioiodine therapy is often used as well, especially if there are any signs of residual disease. Regardless of the size of the cancer and type of operation (lobectomy or some type of thyroidectomy), thyroid hormone therapy is given after surgery. If radioactive iodine treatment is planned, the start of thyroid hormone therapy may be delayed until the treatment is finished (usually about 6 weeks after surgery).

Some doctors recommend central compartment neck dissection (surgical removal of lymph nodes next to the thyroid). Although this operation has not been shown to improve cancer survival, it lowers the risk of cancer coming back in the neck area (**local recurrence**). It also makes it easier to accurately stage the cancer.

Stages II to IV: Most patients have a near-total thyroidectomy or total thyroidectomy with removal and microscopic examination of nearby lymph nodes. Sentinel lymph node biopsy is sometimes done, but this procedure is not yet standard. Some doctors recommend central compartment neck dissection. Although this operation has not been shown to improve survival, it lowers the risk of local recurrence (cancer coming back in the neck area). It also makes it easier to accurately stage the cancer. If cancer has spread to other neck lymph nodes, a modified radical neck dissection (a more extensive surgical removal of lymph nodes from the neck) is often done.

Radioiodine therapy is often used to destroy any remaining thyroid tissue after surgery and to treat any undetectable cancer remaining in the neck or elsewhere in the body that takes up iodine. External beam radiation may be used for cancers that do not take up iodine. Thyroid hormone therapy is used as well.

Recurrent cancer: For cancer that comes back after initial therapy, treatment depends mainly on where the cancer is, although other factors may be important as well. If the cancer recurrence can be located and appears to be resectable (removable), surgery is often used. If the cancer shows up on a radioiodine scan (meaning the cells are taking up iodine), radioiodine therapy may be used, either alone or with surgery. If the cancer does not show up on the scan but is found by other imaging tests such as an MRI scan, external beam radiation may be used. Chemotherapy may be tried if the cancer has spread to several places (and radioiodine treatment is not helpful), although doctors are still trying to find effective drugs for this disease. Another option is taking part in a clinical trial of newer treatments.

Follicular and Hürthle Cell Carcinoma

Stages I to IV: Most doctors recommend near-total or total thyroidectomy for these types of thyroid cancer. This surgery makes radioiodine treatment afterward more effective. In rare cases, a lobectomy of the involved side of the thyroid may be done instead for small cancers. As with papillary cancer, some lymph nodes usually are removed and examined. If cancer has spread to lymph nodes, a central compartment or modified radical neck dissection (surgical removal of lymph nodes from the neck) may be done. Because the thyroid gland is removed, patients will need thyroid hormone therapy as well.

Radioiodine scanning is usually done after surgery to look for areas still taking up iodine. Spread to nearby lymph nodes and to distant sites can be treated by radioiodine therapy. For cancers that don't take up iodine, external beam radiation therapy may help treat the tumor or prevent it from growing back in the neck. Distant metastases may need to be treated with external beam radiation therapy or chemotherapy if they do not respond to radioiodine therapy.

Recurrent cancer: The options for treating cancer that comes back after initial treatment are basically the same as they are for recurrent papillary cancer (see page 63).

Medullary Thyroid Carcinoma

Most doctors advise that patients with an MTC diagnosis be tested for other tumors that are typically seen in patients with the MEN 2 syndromes (see "What Are the Risk Factors for Thyroid Cancer?" on page 13), such as pheochromocytoma and parathyroid adenoma. Screening for pheochromocytoma is particularly important, since the unknown presence of this tumor can make anesthesia and surgery extremely dangerous. If they are forewarned, surgeons and anesthesiologists can medically pretreat the patient to make surgery safer.

Stages I and II: Total thyroidectomy is the main treatment for MTC and often cures patients with stage I or stage II MTC. Regional lymph nodes are usually removed as well (central compartment or modified radical neck dissection). Thyroid hormone therapy is always given, since after total thyroidectomy the patient will not be able to make enough thyroid hormone to stay healthy. Although thyroid hormone therapy reduces the risk of papillary and follicular cancer recurrence, it does not reduce the likelihood of MTC recurrence. Because MTC cells do not take up radioactive iodine, there is no role for radioiodine therapy in treating MTC. Still, some doctors advise giving a dose of radioactive iodine to destroy any remaining normal thyroid tissue. If MTC cells are in or near the thyroid gland, this treatment may affect them as well.

Stages III and IV: Surgery is the same as for stages I and II (usually after screening for MEN 2 syndrome and pheochromocytoma). Thyroid hormone therapy is given afterward. When the tumor is extensive and invades many nearby tissues or cannot be completely removed, external beam radiation therapy may reduce the chance for recurrence in the neck.

Recurrent cancer: Surgery, external beam radiation therapy, or chemotherapy may be needed to treat recurrent disease in the neck or elsewhere. Clinical trials of new treatments may be another option if standard treatments aren't effective.

Genetic testing in MTC: If you are told that you have MTC, even if you are the first one in the family to be diagnosed with this disease, ask your doctor about genetic counseling and testing. Genetic testing can find mutations in the *RET* gene—seen in cases of familial MTC and the MEN 2 syndromes. If you have one of these mutations, it's important that family members (children, brothers, and sisters) be tested as well. Because almost all children and adults with positive genetic test results will have MTC develop at some time, doctors generally agree that thyroidectomy to prevent MTC should be done soon after positive testing, even in children. Some would say *especially* in children, since some hereditary forms of MTC affect children and preteens. Total thyroidectomy can indeed prevent this cancer in carriers who have not yet had it develop. Of course, this means that lifelong thyroid hormone replacement will be needed.

Anaplastic Carcinoma

Stage IV (Note: all anaplastic thyroid cancers are classified as stage IV): Surgery may or may not be used to treat this cancer, because it is often widespread at the time of diagnosis. If the cancer is confined to the local area around the thyroid gland, which is rare, total thyroidectomy may be done. The goal of surgery is to remove as much cancer as possible in the neck area, ideally leaving no cancer tissue behind. Because of the way anaplastic carcinoma spreads, this goal is often difficult or even impossible. Local spread to essential structures within the neck (the windpipe, arteries, etc.) is responsible for most deaths from this type of thyroid cancer.

External beam radiation therapy, alone or combined with chemotherapy, may be used in the following ways:

- to treat the disease before surgery in order to increase the chance of complete tumor removal

- after surgery to try to control any disease that remains in the neck
- in cases where the tumor is too large or widespread to be treated by surgery

If the cancer is causing (or may eventually cause) trouble breathing, a hole (**tracheostomy**) may be placed surgically in the front of the neck to bypass the tumor and allow the patient to breathe more comfortably.

For cancers that have spread to distant sites, chemotherapy may be used, sometimes along with radiation therapy if the cancer is not too widespread. Clinical trials of newer treatments are an option as well.

Your Medical Team

Your **cancer care team** comprises several people, each with a different type of expertise to contribute to your care. One of your team members will take the lead in coordinating your care. Most thyroid cancer patients choose a medical oncologist or endocrinologist to lead the team. It should be clear to all team members who is in charge, and that person should inform the others of your progress.

This alphabetical list will acquaint you with the health care professionals you may encounter, depending on which treatment option and follow-up path you choose, and their areas of expertise:

Anesthesiologist

An anesthesiologist is a medical doctor who administers anesthesia (drugs or gases) to make you

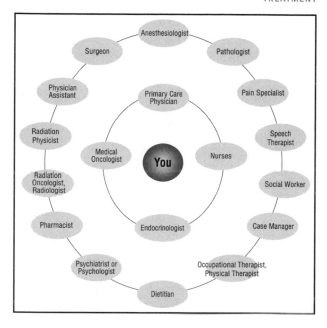

sleep and be unconscious or to prevent or relieve pain during and after a surgical procedure.

Case Manager

The case manager is usually a nurse or oncology nurse specialist, who coordinates the patient's care throughout diagnosis, treatment, and recovery. The case manager provides guidance through the complex health care system by cutting through red tape, getting responses to questions, managing crises, and connecting the patient and family to needed resources.

Dietitian

A dietitian is specially trained to help you make healthy diet choices and maintain a healthy weight before, during, and after treatment. Dietitians can help patients deal with side effects of treatment, such as nausea, vomiting, or sore throat. A registered dietitian (RD) has at least a bachelor's degree and has passed a national competency exam.

Endocrinologist

An endocrinologist is a doctor who specializes in the diagnosis and treatment of disorders of the endocrine (hormone) system.

Medical Oncologist

A medical oncologist (also sometimes called an oncologist) is a medical doctor you may see after diagnosis. The oncologist is a cancer expert who understands specific types of cancer, their treatments, and their causes. He or she may help cancer patients make decisions about a course of treatment and then manage all phases of cancer care. Oncologists most often become involved when you need chemotherapy, but can also prescribe hormonal therapy and other anticancer drugs.

Nurses

During your treatment you will be in contact with different types of nurses.

Clinical nurse specialist: A clinical nurse specialist (CSN) is a nurse who has a master's degree in a specific area, such as oncology, psychiatry, or critical care nursing. The CSN often provides expertise to staff and may provide special services to patients, such as leading support groups and coordinating cancer care.

Nurse practitioner: A nurse practitioner is a registered nurse with a master's degree or doctoral degree who can manage the care of patients with thyroid cancer and has additional training in primary care. He or she shares many tasks with your doctors, such as recording your medical history, conducting physical examinations, and doing follow-up care. In most states, a nurse practitioner can prescribe medications with a doctor's supervision.

Oncology-certified nurse: An oncology-certified nurse is a registered nurse who has demonstrated an in-depth knowledge of oncology care. He or she has passed a certification examination. Oncology-certified nurses are found in all areas of cancer practice.

Registered nurse: A registered nurse has an associate or bachelor's degree in nursing and has passed a state licensing exam. He or she can monitor your condition, provide treatment, educate you about side effects, and help you adjust to cancer, both physically and emotionally.

Occupational Therapist

An occupational therapist is a health care professional who helps restore self care, work, or leisure skills. They generally have a 4-year degree and are certified.

Pain Specialist

Pain specialists are doctors, nurses, and pharmacists who are experts in managing pain. They can help you find pain control methods that are effective and allow you to maintain your quality of life. Not all doctors and nurses are trained in pain care, so you may have to request a pain specialist if your pain relief needs are not being met.

Pathologist

A pathologist is a medical doctor specially trained in diagnosing disease based on examination of microscopic tissue and fluid samples. He or she will determine the classification (cell type) of your cancer, help determine the stage (extent) and grade (estimate of aggressiveness) of your cancer, and issue a pathology report so that you and your doctor can decide on treatment options.

Personal or Primary Care Physician

A personal physician may be a general doctor, internist, or family practice doctor. He or she is often the medical doctor you first saw when you noticed symptoms of illness. This general or family practice doctor may be a member of your medical team, but a specialist is most often a patient's cancer care team leader.

Pharmacist

A pharmacist is a health professional who dispenses medications and counsels people on their proper use and potential adverse side effects. Pharmacists participate in disease management in collaboration with physicians and other health professionals.

Physical Therapist

A physical therapist is a health professional who helps restore, maintain, and promote overall fitness and health.

Physician Assistant

Physicians assistants (PAs) are health care professionals licensed to practice medicine with physician supervision. Physician assistants practice in the areas of primary care medicine (family medicine, internal medicine, pediatrics, and obstetrics and gynecology) as well as in surgery and the surgical subspecialties. Under the supervision of a doctor, they can diagnose and treat medical problems and, in most states, can also prescribe medications.

Psychologist or Psychiatrist

A psychologist is a licensed mental health professional who is often part of the cancer care team. He or she provides counseling on emotional and psychological issues. A psychologist may have specialized training and experience in treating people with cancer.

A psychiatrist is a medical doctor specializing in mental health and behavioral disorders. Psychiatrists provide counseling and can also prescribe medications.

Radiation Oncologist

A radiation oncologist is a medical doctor who specializes in treating cancer by using therapeutic radiation (high-energy x-rays or seeds). If you choose radiation, the radiation oncologist evaluates you frequently during the course of treatment and at intervals afterward. The radiation oncologist will usually work closely with your oncologist and will help you make decisions about radiation therapy options. A radiation oncologist is assisted by a radiation therapist during treatment and works with a radiation physicist, an expert who is trained in ensuring that you receive the correct dose of radiation treatment. The physicist is also assisted by a dosimetrist, a technician who helps plan and calculate the dosage, number, and length of your radiation treatments.

Radiation Physicist

A radiation physicist ensures that the radiation machine delivers the right amount of radiation to the correct site in the body. The physicist works with the radiation oncologist to choose the treatment schedule and dose that will have the best chance of killing the most cancer cells.

Radiologist

A radiologist is a medical doctor specializing in the use of imaging procedures (for example, diagnostic x-rays, ultrasound, magnetic resonance images, and bone scans) that produce pictures of internal body structures. He or she has special training in diagnosing cancer and other diseases and interpreting the results of imaging procedures. Your radiologist issues a radiology report describing the findings to your endocrinologist, or radiation oncologist. The radiology images and report may be used to aid in diagnosis; to help classify and determine the extent of your illness; to help locate tumors during procedures, surgery, and radiation treatment; or to look for the possible spread or recurrence of the cancer after treatment.

Social Worker

A social worker is a health specialist, usually with a master's degree, who is licensed or certified by the state in which he or she works. A social worker is an expert in coordinating and providing social services. He or she is trained to help you and your family deal with a range of emotional and practical challenges, such as finances, child care, emotional issues, family concerns and relationships, transportation, and problems with the health care system. If your social worker is trained in cancer-related problems, he or she can counsel you about your fears or concerns, help answer questions about diagnosis and treatment, and lead cancer support groups. You may communicate with your social worker during a hospital stay or on an outpatient basis.

Speech Therapist

A speech therapist is a health professional who addresses a person's speech production, vocal production, and swallowing difficulties.

Surgeon

Several different types of surgeons provide treatment for thyroid cancer. A general surgeon is trained to operate on all parts of the body, including the endocrine system.

A surgical oncologist is a surgeon who has had advanced training in the surgical treatment of people with cancer. Cancer centers usually have one or more such individuals on their staff. A head and neck surgeon is a surgeon who has had advanced training in the surgical treatment of people with endocrine system disorders or diseases.

Although each type of surgeon has a different area of expertise, each plays the same role in treating people with thyroid cancer. If you require surgery as part of your treatment, the surgeon will perform the operation and then manage any side effects you might have. He or she will also issue a report to your other doctors to help determine the rest of your treatment plan.

More Treatment Information

For more details on treatment options—including some that may not be addressed in this book—the National Comprehensive Cancer Network (NCCN) and the National Cancer Institute (NCI) are good sources of information.

The NCCN, made up of experts from many of the nation's leading cancer centers, develops cancer treatment guidelines for doctors to use when treating patients. Those guidelines are available on the NCCN Web site (**www.nccn.org**).

The NCI provides treatment information via telephone (**800-4-CANCER**) and its Web site (**www.cancer.gov**). Information for patients, as well as more detailed information intended for use by cancer care professionals, is also available on **www.cancer.gov.**

Questions to Ask

What Should You Ask Your Doctor About Thyroid Cancer?

As you deal with your thyroid cancer and the process of treatment, you need to have honest, open discussions with your cancer care team. You should feel free to ask any question that is on your mind, no matter how minor it might seem. Consider these questions:

- What kind of thyroid cancer do I have?
- Are there tests that need to be done before treatment?
- Has my cancer spread beyond the thyroid gland?
- What is the stage of my thyroid cancer? What does this mean in my case?
- Is this form of thyroid cancer hereditary? Should my family be tested?
- How much surgery do I need? Should I get other treatments as well?
- What should I do to be ready for treatment?
- Will I need to take thyroid hormone for the rest of my life?

- Have you performed many operations on the thyroid?
- How do you feel about sentinel lymph node biopsy in my case?
- What other treatment choices do I have?
- What side effects can I expect from my treatments?
- What are the other risks of treatments?
- How long will it take me to recover from treatment?
- When can I go back to work after treatment?
- How soon after treatment can I have sex?
- Will this treatment affect my ability to have children? Do I need to avoid pregnancy for awhile?
- What type of follow-up will I need after treatment?
- What are the chances that my cancer will recur?
- Should I get a second opinion?
- Based on what you've learned about my cancer, what are my chances of being cured?

You will no doubt have other questions about your own personal situation. Be sure to write down your questions so that you remember to ask them during each visit with your cancer care team. For example, you may want to ask about clinical trials you may be eligible for. Keep in mind, too, that doctors are not the only ones who can provide you with information. Other health care professionals, such as nurses and social workers, may have the answers you seek.

After Treatment

What Happens After Treatment for Thyroid Cancer?

Completing treatment can be both stressful and exciting. You will be relieved to finish treatment, yet it is hard not to worry about cancer coming back. (When cancer returns, it is called recurrence.) Fear of recurrence is a common concern among those who have had cancer. It may take awhile before your confidence in your own recovery begins to feel real and your fears are somewhat relieved. Even with no recurrences, people who have had cancer learn to live with uncertainty.

Follow-up Care

After your treatment is over, it is very important to keep all follow-up appointments. During these visits, your doctors will ask about symptoms, examine you, and possibly order blood tests or imaging tests such as radioiodine scans or CT scans. Follow-up is needed to check for cancer recurrence or spread, as well as possible side effects of certain treatments. This is the time for you to ask your cancer care team any questions you need answered and to discuss any concerns you might have. Because most people do very well after treatment, follow-up care can continue for a lifetime. Follow-up care is very important since thyroid cancers grow slowly and can recur even 10 to 20 years after initial treatment. Your cancer care team will explain what tests you need and how often they should be done.

If you have had a papillary *or* follicular cancer, and your thyroid gland has been completely removed and ablated (destroyed), your doctors will do at least 1 radioiodine scan after your initial treatment is complete. This scan is usually done about 6 to 12 months later. After that, if the scan results are negative, then you will generally not need further scans unless indicated by other studies or findings. Your blood will also be tested for thyroglobulin. This substance is made by thyroid tissue and, after total thyroid removal and **ablation,** should be absent from your blood. If thyroglobulin begins to appear, it may be a sign the cancer is coming back, and further testing will be done. This process usually includes a radioactive iodine scan, and may include PET scans and other imaging tests. For those with a low-risk, small papillary cancer that was treated by removing only one lobe of the thyroid, a physical examination by your doctor, as well as a thyroid ultrasound and periodic chest x-ray, is typical.

Treatment of recurrent cancer is described in the section "How Is Thyroid Cancer Treated?" on page 41.

If you had MTC, your doctors will check your blood levels of calcitonin and carcinoembryonic antigen (CEA). If these begin to rise, imaging tests such as a CT or MRI scan will be done to look for any cancer that may be coming back. If the tests show recurrent cancer, treatment is as described in the section, "How Is Thyroid Cancer Treated?" on page 41.

Each type of treatment for thyroid cancer has side effects that may last for a few months. Some, like the need for oral thyroid hormone, may be permanent. You may be able to hasten your recovery by being aware of the side effects before you start treatment. You might be able to take steps to reduce them and shorten the length of time they last. Don't hesitate to tell your cancer care team about any symptoms or side effects that bother you so they can help you manage them.

Seeing a New Doctor

At some point after your cancer diagnosis and treatment, you may find yourself in the office of a new doctor. Your original doctor may have moved or retired, or you may have moved or changed doctors for some reason. It is important that you be able to give your new doctor the exact details of your diagnosis and treatment. Make sure you have the following information handy:

- a copy of your pathology report from any biopsy or surgery
- if you had surgery, a copy of your operative report

- if you were hospitalized, a copy of the discharge summary that every doctor must prepare when patients are sent home from the hospital
- finally, since some drugs can have long-term side effects, a list of your drugs, drug doses, and when you took them

It is also important to keep medical insurance. Even though no one wants to think of the cancer coming back, it is always a possibility. If it happens, the last thing you want is to have to worry about paying for treatment.

Lifestyle Changes to Consider During and After Treatment

Having cancer and dealing with treatment can be time-consuming and emotionally draining, but it can also be a time to look at your life in new ways. Maybe you are thinking about how to improve your health over the long term. Some people even begin this process during cancer treatment.

Make Healthier Choices

Think about what your life was like before you found out you had cancer. Were there things you did that might have made you less healthy? Maybe you drank too much alcohol, ate more than you needed, smoked, or didn't exercise very often. Emotionally, maybe you kept your feelings bottled up, or maybe you let stressful situations go on too long.

Now is not the time to feel guilty or to blame yourself. However, you can start making changes today that can have positive effects for the rest of your life. Not only will you feel better, you will also be healthier. What better time than now to take advantage of the motivation you have as a result of going through a life-changing experience like having cancer? You can start by working on those things that you feel most concerned about. Get help with those that are harder for you. For instance, if you are thinking about quitting smoking and need help, call the American Cancer Society's Quitline® tobacco cessation program at **800-ACS-2345.**

Diet and Nutrition

Eating right can be a challenge for anyone, but it can get even tougher during and after cancer treatment. For instance, treatment often may change your sense of taste. Nausea can be a problem. You may lose your appetite for awhile and lose weight when you don't want to. On the other hand, some people gain weight even without eating more. This experience can be frustrating, too.

If you are losing weight or have taste problems during treatment, do the best you can with eating and remember that these problems usually improve over time. You may want to ask your cancer care team for a referral to a dietitian, an expert in nutrition who can help you deal with some of the side effects of your treatment. You may also find it helps to eat small portions of food every 2 to 3 hours until you feel better and can go back to a more normal schedule.

One of the best things you can do after treatment is to put healthy eating habits in place. You will be surprised at the long-term benefits of some simple changes, like increasing the variety of healthy foods you eat. Try to eat 5 or more servings of vegetables and fruits each day. Choose whole grain foods instead of white flour and sugars. Try to limit meats that are high in fat. Cut back on processed meats like hot dogs, bologna, and bacon. Get rid of them altogether if you can. If you drink alcohol, limit yourself to 1 or 2 drinks a day at the most. And don't forget to get some type of regular exercise. The combination of a good diet and regular exercise will help you maintain a healthy weight and keep you feeling more energetic.

Rest, Fatigue, Work, and Exercise

Fatigue is a very common symptom in people being treated for cancer. This fatigue is often not an ordinary type of tiredness but a "bone-weary" exhaustion that doesn't get better with rest. For some, this fatigue lasts a long time after treatment and can discourage them from physical activity. However, exercise can actually help you reduce fatigue. Studies have shown that patients who follow an exercise program tailored to their personal needs feel physically and emotionally improved and can cope better.

If you are ill and need to be on bed rest during treatment, it is normal to expect your fitness, endurance, and muscle strength to decline some. Physical therapy can help you maintain strength and range of motion in your muscles, which can help fight fatigue and the sense of depression that sometimes comes with feeling so tired. Any program of physical activity should fit your own situation. An older person who has never exercised will not be able to take on the same amount of exercise as a 20-year-old person who plays tennis 3 times a week. If you haven't exercised in a few years but can still get around, you may want to think about taking short walks.

Talk with your cancer care team before starting an exercise program, and get their opinion about your exercise plans. Then, try to get an exercise buddy so that you're not doing it alone. Having family or friends involved when starting a new exercise program can give you that extra boost of support to keep you going when the push just isn't there.

If you are very tired, though, you will need to balance activity with rest. It is okay to rest when you need to. It is really hard for some people to allow themselves to do that when they are used to working all day or taking care of a household.

For more information about fatigue, please see our fatigue and anemia information, which can be ordered by calling **800-ACS-2345,** or view the information at **www.cancer.org.**

Exercise can improve your physical and emotional health.

- It improves your cardiovascular fitness (heart and circulation).
- It strengthens your muscles.
- It reduces fatigue.
- It lowers anxiety and depression.
- It makes you feel generally happier.
- It helps you feel better about yourself.

We know that over the long term, exercise plays a role in preventing some cancers. The American Cancer Society, in its guidelines on physical activity for cancer prevention, recommends that adults take part in at least 30 minutes of moderate to vigorous physical activity, above usual activities, on 5 or more days of the week; 45 to 60 minutes of intentional physical activity are preferable. Children and teens are encouraged to try for at least 60 minutes a day of moderate to vigorous physical activity on at least 5 days a week.

How About Your Emotional Health?

Once your treatment ends, you may find yourself overwhelmed by emotions. This reaction happens to a lot of people. You may have been going through so much during treatment that you could focus only on getting through your treatment. Now you may find that you think about the potential of your own death, or the effect of your cancer on your family, friends, and career. You may also begin to reevaluate your relationship with your spouse or partner. Unexpected issues may also cause concern—for instance, as you become healthier and have fewer doctor visits, you will see your cancer care team less often. Having fewer check-ups can be a source of anxiety for some.

This is an ideal time to seek out emotional and social support. You need people you can turn to for strength and comfort. Support can come in many forms: family, friends, cancer support groups, church or spiritual groups, online support communities, or individual counselors.

Almost everyone who has been through cancer can benefit from getting some type of support. What's best for you depends on your situation and personality. Some people feel safe in peer-support groups or education groups. Others would rather talk in an informal setting, such as church. Others may feel more at ease talking one-on-one with a trusted friend or counselor. Whatever your source of strength or comfort may be, make sure you have a place to go with your concerns.

The cancer journey can feel very lonely. It is not necessary or realistic to try to do everything by yourself and make all the decisions about your care. Your friends and family may feel shut out if you decide not to include them. Let them in—and let in anyone else who you feel may help.

If you aren't sure who can help, call your American Cancer Society at **800-ACS-2345,** and we can put you in touch with an appropriate group or resource. You can't change the fact that you have had cancer. What you can change is how you live the rest of your life—making healthy choices and feeling as well as possible, physically and emotionally.

What Happens if Treatment Is No Longer Working?

If cancer continues to grow after one kind of treatment, or if it returns, it is often possible to try another treatment plan that might still cure the cancer, or at least shrink the tumors enough to help you live longer and feel better. On the other hand, when a person has received several different medical treatments and the cancer has not been cured, over time the cancer tends to become resistant to all treatment. At this time, it's important to weigh the possible limited benefit of a new treatment against the possible downsides, including continued doctor visits and treatment side effects.

Everyone has his or her own way of looking at this situation. Some people may want to focus on remaining comfortable during their limited time left. This point is likely to be the most difficult time in your battle with cancer—when you have tried everything medically within reason and it's just not working anymore. Although your doctor may offer you new treatment, you need to consider that at some point, continuing treatment is not likely to improve your health or change your prognosis or survival.

If you want to continue treatment to fight your cancer as long as you can, you still need to consider the odds of more treatment having any benefit. In many cases, your doctor can estimate the response rate for the treatment you are considering. Some people are tempted to try more chemotherapy or radiation, for example, even when their doctors say that the odds of benefit are less than 1%. In this situation, you need to think about and understand your reasons for choosing this plan. No matter what you decide to do, it is important that you be as comfortable as possible. Make sure you are asking for and getting treatment for any symptoms you might have, such as pain. This type of treatment is called palliative treatment.

Palliative treatment helps relieve these symptoms, but is not expected to cure the disease; its main purpose is to improve your **quality of life.** Sometimes, the treatments you get to control your symptoms are similar to the treatments used to treat cancer. For example, radiation therapy might be given to help relieve pain from metastasis. Or chemotherapy might be given to help shrink a tumor and keep it from causing shortness of breath. But this is not the same as receiving treatment to try to cure the cancer.

At some point, you may benefit from hospice care. Most of the time, hospice care can be given at home. Your cancer may be causing symptoms or problems that need attention, and hospice focuses on your comfort. You should know that receiving hospice care doesn't mean you can't have treatment for the problems caused by your cancer or other health conditions. It just means that the focus of your care is on living life as fully as possible and feeling as well as you can at this difficult stage of your cancer.

Remember also that maintaining hope is important. Your hope for a cure may not be as bright, but there is still hope for good times with family and friends—times that are filled with happiness and meaning. In a way, pausing at this time in your cancer treatment is an opportunity to refocus on the most important things in your life. Now is the time to do some things you've always wanted to do and to stop doing the things you no longer want to do.

Latest Research

What's New in Thyroid Cancer Research and Treatment?

Important research into thyroid cancer is under way right now in many university hospitals, medical centers, and other institutions around the country. Each year, scientists find out more about what causes the disease, how to prevent it, and how to improve treatment. In past years, for example, evidence has grown showing the benefits of combining surgery with radioactive iodine therapy and thyroid hormone therapy. The results include higher cure rates, lower recurrence rates, and longer survival.

Genetics

Recent identification of the genetic causes of familial (inherited) MTC now makes it possible to identify family members carrying the abnormal gene and to prevent cancer from developing. Researchers are optimistic that progress in understanding the abnormal genes that cause sporadic (not inherited) thyroid cancer, especially papillary cancer, will eventually lead to better treatments.

Treatment

New treatments for thyroid cancer are being tested in several types of clinical trials.

Chemotherapy

Some studies are testing the value of newer chemotherapy drugs such as paclitaxel (Taxol) and other drugs, as well as combined chemotherapy and radiation in treating anaplastic thyroid cancer.

Targeted Therapies

In general, thyroid cancers have not responded well to chemotherapy. But exciting data are emerging about some newer targeted drugs. Unlike standard chemotherapy drugs, which work by attacking rapidly growing cells in general (which includes cancer cells), these drugs attack specific targets on cancer cells.

Tyrosine kinase inhibitors: A class of targeted drugs known as **tyrosine kinase inhibitors** has already been used successfully to treat some other forms of cancer. These drugs may help reverse the abnormal growth of thyroid cancer cells that results from mutations of certain genes, such as *BRAF* and *RET/PTC*. Some of the tyrosine kinase inhibitors being tested against thyroid cancer in clinical trials include sorafenib (Nexavar), sunitinib (Sutent), motesanib (AMG 706), and axitinib (AG-013736). Early, small studies have shown some promising results, but more research is needed before these drugs are routinely used for thyroid cancer.

Antiangiogenesis drugs: As tumors grow, they need a larger blood supply to get enough nutrients.

They do this by causing new blood vessels to form (a process called **angiogenesis**). Antiangiogenesis drugs work by disrupting these new blood vessels. Some of the tyrosine kinase inhibitors listed above have antiangiogenic properties. Another drug with these properties is combretastatin A-4 phosphate (CA4P), which has shown some promising early results and is now being tested in larger studies.

Monoclonal antibodies: Monoclonal antibodies are man-made versions of immune system proteins designed to attack a specific target. Studies are testing radiolabeled monoclonal antibodies (antibodies with radioactive material attached) for treating MTC. CEA is a protein that is not normally found in adult tissues. But many MTCs make CEA. Since radioiodine treatment is not useful in MTC because MTC does not take up iodine, the ability to deliver radiation (and other treatments) to MTC cells by bonding radioactive material to anti-CEA antibodies appears promising. Studies of this technique are in progress.

Resources

The American Cancer Society is happy to address any cancer-related topic. If you have any questions, please call us at **800-ACS-2345**, 24 hours a day.

More Information from Your American Cancer Society

The following related materials may be ordered through our toll-free number: **800-ACS-2345 (800-227-2345)**.

Spanish language versions of these documents are also available.

After Diagnosis: A Guide for Patients and Families

Home Care for the Person with Cancer: A Guide for Patients and Families

Understanding Chemotherapy: A Guide for Patients and Families

Understanding Radiation Therapy: A Guide for Patients and Families

National Organizations and Web Sites

In addition to the American Cancer Society, the following other sources of patient information and support are available*:

Inclusion on this list does not imply endorsement by the American Cancer Society.

American Association of Clinical Endocrinologists
Telephone: 904-353-7878
Internet address: www.aace.com

American Thyroid Association
Toll-free number: 800-THYROID
Internet address: www.thyroid.org

Endocrine Web
Internet address: www.endocrineweb.com

National Cancer Institute
Toll-free number: 800-4-CANCER (800-422-6237)
Internet address: www.cancer.gov

ThyCa: Thyroid Cancer Survivor's Association
Toll-free number: 877-588-7904
Internet address: www.thyca.org

Thyroid Foundation of America
Toll-free number: 800-832-8321
Internet address: www.allthyroid.org

References

American Cancer Society. *Cancer Facts & Figures 2008*.
Atlanta, GA: American Cancer Society; 2008.

American Joint Committee on Cancer. Thyroid. In:
Greene FL, Page DL, Fleming ID, Fritz A, Balch
CM, Haller DG, Morrow M, eds. *AJCC Cancer
Staging Manual*. 6th ed. New York: Springer;
2002:77–87.

Baudin E, Schlumberger M. New therapeutic
approaches for metastatic thyroid carcinoma. *Lancet
Oncol*. 2007;8(2):148–156.

Carling T, Udelsman R. Thyroid tumors. In: DeVita VT,
Hellman S, Rosenberg SA, eds. *Cancer: Principles
and Practice of Oncology*. 7th ed. Philadelphia, PA:
Lippincott Williams & Wilkins; 2005:1502–1520.

Davies L, Welch HG. Increasing incidence of thyroid
cancer in the United States, 1973-2002. *JAMA*.
2006;295(18):2164–2167.

Fagin JA. Challenging dogma in thyroid cancer molecular genetics—role of RET/PTC and BRAF in tumor initiation. *J Clin Endocrinol Metab.* 2004;89(9):4264–4266.

Frates MC, Benson CB, Charboneau IW, et al. Management of thyroid nodules detected at US: Society of Radiologists in Ultrasound consensus conference statement. *Radiology.* 2005;237(3):794–800.

Hundahl SA, Cady B, Cunningham MP, et al. Initial results from a prospective cohort study of 5583 cases of thyroid carcinoma treated in the United States during 1996. An American College of Surgeons Commission on Cancer patient care evaluation study. *Cancer.* 2000;89(1):202–217.

National Cancer Institute. Cancer Topics Physician Data Query (PDQ) Web site. Thyroid cancer treatment (PDQ). 2007. National Cancer Institute Web site. http://www.cancer.gov/cancertopics/pdq/treatment/thyroid/healthprofessional. Accessed August 16, 2007.

National Cancer Institute. Contents of the SEER Cancer Statistics Review, 1975–2004. 2007. Surveillance Epidemiology and End Results (SEER) Web site. http://seer.cancer.gov/csr/1975_2004/sections.html. Accessed August 16, 2007.

National Comprehensive Cancer Network. NCCN Clinical Practice Guidelines in Oncology: Thyroid Carcinoma. V.2.2007. National Comprehensive Cancer Network Web site. http://www.nccn.org/professionals/physician_gls/PDF/thyroid.pdf. Accessed August 16, 2007.

Sherman SI. Thyroid carcinoma. *Lancet.* 2003; 361(9356):501–511.

Weber T, Schilling T, Buchler MW. Thyroid carcinoma. *Curr Opin Oncol.* 2006;18(1):30–35.

Wiegel RJ, Macdonald JS, Haller D, McDougall IR. Cancer of the endocrine system. In: Abeloff MD, Armitage JO, Niederhuber JE, Kastan MB, McKenna WG, eds. *Clinical Oncology.* 3rd ed. Philadelphia, PA: Elsevier; 2004:1611–1648.

Glossary

ablation (a-BLAY-shun): the destruction or removal of a body part or tissue or its function by use of surgery, hormones, extreme hot or cold temperatures, drugs, radiation, or other methods.

adenocarcinoma (add-uh-no-kahr-si-NO-muh): cancer of the glandular cells.

adenoma (add-uh-NO-muh): a noncancerous tumor.

AJCC staging system: *see* American Joint Committee on Cancer staging system.

alternative medicine (alternative therapy): an unproven medication or therapy that is recommended instead of standard (proven) therapy. Some alternative therapies have dangerous or even life-threatening side effects. With others, the main danger is that the patient may lose the opportunity to benefit from standard therapy. The American Cancer Society recommends that patients considering the use of any alternative or complementary therapies discuss them with their cancer care team. *See also* unproven therapy. *Compare with* complementary medicine, standard therapy.

American Joint Committee on Cancer (AJCC) TNM staging system: a system for describing the extent of a cancer's spread by using Roman numerals from 0 through IV. Also called the TNM system. *See also* staging.

anaplastic carcinoma (A-nuh-PLAS-tik kahr-si-NO-muh): a rare type of carcinoma of the thyroid gland, with the potential to become highly malignant and locally invasive. Also called undifferentiated carcinoma of the thyroid gland, its cellular pattern is atypical.

anesthesia (an-es-THEE-zhuh): the loss of feeling or sensation as a result of drugs or gases. **General anesthesia** causes loss of consciousness (puts you to sleep). **Local** or **regional anesthesia** numbs only a certain area of the body. *See also* anesthetic.

anesthetic (an-es-THEH-tik): a topical or intravenous substance that causes loss of feeling or awareness in a part of the body. General anesthetics are used to put patients to sleep for procedures. *See also* anesthesia.

angiogenesis (an-jee-o-JEN-uh-sis): the formation of new blood vessels. Some cancer treatments work by blocking angiogenesis, thus preventing blood from reaching the tumor.

antibody: a protein produced by the body's immune system cells and released into the blood. Antibodies defend the body against foreign agents, such as bacteria. These agents contain certain substances called antigens. Each antibody works against a specific antigen.

benign: not cancer; not malignant.

biopsy (BUY-op-see): the removal of a sample of tissue to see whether cancer cells are present. There are several kinds of biopsies. In an endoscopic biopsy, a small sample of tissue is removed by using instruments operated through an endoscope or tube into the area of concern. *See also* fine needle aspiration, CT–guided needle biopsy.

brachytherapy (brake-ee-THER-uh-pee): internal radiation treatment given by placing radioactive seeds or pellets directly into the tumor or close to it. Also called interstitial radiation therapy or seed implantation.

calcitonin (KAL-sih-TOH-nin): a thyroid hormone produced by the C cells of the thyroid gland, which helps regulate calcium levels in the blood.

cancer: cancer is not just one disease but a group of diseases. All forms of cancer cause cells in the body to change and grow out of control. Most types of cancer cells form a lump or mass called a tumor. The tumor can invade and destroy healthy tissue. Cells from the tumor can break away and travel to other parts of the body. There they can continue to grow. This spreading process is called metastasis. When cancer spreads, it is still named after the part of the body where it started. For example, if breast cancer spreads to the lungs, it is still called breast cancer, not lung cancer.

Some cancers, such as blood cancers, do not form a tumor. Not all tumors are cancer. Another word for cancerous is malignant. A tumor that is not cancer is called benign. Benign tumors do not grow and spread the way cancer does. Benign tumors are usually not a threat to life.

cancer care team: the group of health care professionals who work together to find, treat, and care for people with cancer. The cancer care team may include the following and others: primary care physicians, pathologists, oncology specialists (medical oncologist, radiation oncologist), surgeons (including surgical specialists such as urologists, gynecologists, and neurosurgeons), nurses, oncology nurse specialists, and oncology social workers. Whether the team is linked formally or informally, there is usually one person who takes the job of coordinating the team.

cancer cell: a cell that divides and reproduces abnormally and has the potential to spread throughout the body, crowding out normal cells and tissue. *See also* metastasis, cancer.

carcinoembryonic antigen (kahr-si-no-em-bre-AHN-ik AN-tuh-jen) (CEA): a substance normally found in fetal tissue. If found in an increased amount in the blood of an adult, it suggests that cancer may be present. It is used as a tumor marker for some thyroid cancers.

carcinoma (kahr-si-NO-muh): any cancerous tumor that begins in the lining layer of organs. At least 80% of all cancers are carcinomas.

cartilage (KAR-tih-lij): fibrous connective tissue that lines the joints and gives structure to various parts of the body, including the nose and ears.

C cells: cells located in the thyroid gland that produce calcitonin, a hormone that maintains a healthy level of calcium in the blood. Situated between or within the walls of the follicles, C cells are also called parafollicular cells. *See also* calcitonin.

CEA: *see* carcinoembryonic antigen.

cell: the basic unit of which all living things are made. Cells replace themselves by splitting and forming new cells (mitosis). The processes that control the formation of new cells and the death of old cells are disrupted in cancer.

central compartment neck dissection (dye-SEK-shun): surgery to remove lymph nodes located near the thyroid gland and other related tissues in the central portion of the neck. *See also* lymph nodes. *Compare with* modified radical neck dissection.

chemotherapy (key-mo-THER-uh-pee): treatment with drugs to destroy cancer cells. Chemotherapy is often used, either alone or with surgery or radiation, to treat cancer that has spread or come back (recurred), or when there is a strong chance that it could recur. *See also* systemic therapy.

clinical trials: research studies to test new drugs or other treatments to compare current, standard treatments with others that may be better. Before a new treatment is used on people, it is studied in the laboratory. If laboratory studies suggest the treatment will work, the next step is to test its value for patients. These human studies are called clinical trials. *See also* control group.

cold nodule: a growth or lump in the thyroid gland that absorbs less radioactivity than the surrounding tissue, as seen during radioiodine scanning. Cold nodules can be benign or malignant. *See also* nodule, radioiodine scan, radioactivity. *Compare with* hot nodule.

colloid: a gelatinous product of the thyroid gland, consisting mainly of thyroglobulin. Colloid is the precursor and storage form of thyroid hormone. *See also* thyroglobulin.

complementary medicine (complementary therapy): treatment used in addition to standard therapy. Some complementary therapies may help relieve certain symptoms of cancer, relieve side effects of standard cancer therapy, or improve a patient's sense of well-being. The American Cancer Society recommends that patients considering the use of any alternative or complementary therapies discuss these therapies with their cancer care team, since many of these treatments are unproven and some can be harmful. *Compare with* alternative medicine.

computed tomography (to-MAHG ruh fee): an imaging test in which many x-rays are taken of a part of the body from different angles. These images are combined by a computer to produce cross-sectional pictures of internal organs. Except for the injection of a contrast dye (needed in some but not all cases), this is a painless procedure that can be done in an outpatient clinic. It is often referred to as "CT" or "CAT" scanning. *Compare with* positron emission tomography (PET).

control group: in research or clinical trials, the group that does not receive the treatment being tested. The group may get a placebo or sham treatment, or it may receive standard therapy. Also called the comparison group. *See also* clinical trials.

Cowden disease: an inherited condition characterized by lesions that form on various organs, especially in the breast, thyroid, colon, skin, oral mucosa, and intestines, and is associated with a higher risk for developing malignancies in the organs involved.

CT–guided needle biopsy (BUY-op-see): a procedure that uses special x-rays to locate a mass, while the radiologist advances a biopsy needle toward it. The images are repeated until the doctor is sure the needle is in the tumor or mass. A small sample of tissue is then taken from the mass to be examined under a microscope. *See also* biopsy.

CT scan or CAT scan: *see* computed tomography.

curative treatment: treatment aimed at producing a cure. *Compare with* palliative treatment.

cyst (sist): a closed cavity in the body filled with fluid or semisolid material.

detection: finding disease. Early detection means that the disease is found at an early stage, before it has grown large or spread to other sites.

diagnosis: identifying a disease by its signs or symptoms and by using imaging procedures and laboratory findings. For some types of cancer, the earlier a diagnosis is made, the better the chance for long-term survival.

differentiated (cells): cells that closely resemble healthy organ tissue cells. In cell differentiation, normal cells go through physical changes to form the different, specialized tissues of the body. *Compare with* undifferentiated cells.

DNA: deoxyribonucleic acid. DNA is the genetic "blueprint" found in the nucleus of each cell. It holds genetic information on cell growth, division, and function.

endocrine (EN-doh-krin) glands: ductless organs that make and release hormones directly into the bloodstream and influence metabolism and other body processes. The pituitary, thyroid, and adrenal glands are all examples of endocrine glands.

external beam radiation therapy (EBRT): radiation that is focused from a source outside the body on the area affected by the cancer. It is much like getting a diagnostic x-ray, but for a longer period.

familial adenomatous polyposis: (fuh-MIL-ee-uhl add-uh-NO-muh-tus pahl-ih-POH-sis) (FAP): an inherited condition that is a risk factor for colorectal cancer. People with this syndrome typically develop hundreds of polyps in the colon and rectum. Usually, one or more of these polyps becomes cancerous if preventive surgery is not done.

familial medullary thyroid carcinoma: an inherited form of medullary thyroid cancer that develops in the C cells of the thyroid gland. *See also* medullary thyroid carcinoma, C cells.

FDA: *see* U.S. Food and Drug Administration.

fine needle aspiration: a procedure in which a thin needle is used to draw up (aspirate) samples for examination under a microscope. *See also* biopsy.

five (5)-year relative survival rate: the percentage of people with a certain cancer who have not died of it within 5 years. This number is different from the 5-year survival rate in that it does not include people who have died of unrelated causes. *Compare with* five (5)-year survival rate.

five (5)-year survival rate: the percentage of people with a given cancer who are expected to survive 5 years or longer with the disease. Five-year survival rates have some drawbacks. Although the rates are based on the most recent information available, they may include data from patients treated several years earlier. Advances in cancer treatment often occur quickly. Five-year survival rates, while statistically valid, may not reflect these advances. They should not be seen as a predictor in an individual case. *Compare with* five (5)-year relative survival rate.

follicular adenocarcinoma: *see* follicular thyroid cancer.

follicular carcinoma: *see* follicular thyroid cancer.

follicular thyroid cancer (fuh-LIH-kyoo-ler THY-royd KAN-ser): a type of cancer that forms in the follicular cells. Thyroid follicles are cystlike structures in the thyroid gland that are filled with a colloid, a stored form of thyroid hormone. *Compare with* medullary thyroid cancer.

gadolinium (GA-duh-LIH-nee-um): a metal element that is used in magnetic resonance imaging (MRI) and other imaging methods. It is a contrast agent that helps reveal abnormal tissue in the body during an imaging procedure.

Gardner syndrome: like familial adenomatous polyposis, Gardner syndrome is an inherited condition that results in colon polyps that develop at a young age and often lead to cancer. Thyroid cancer may also occur. Gardner syndrome can also cause benign (noncancerous) tumors of the skin, soft connective tissue, and bones.

gene: a segment of DNA that contains information on hereditary characteristics such as hair color, eye color, and height, as well as susceptibility to certain diseases. *See also* DNA, genetic risk factor, genetic counseling, genetic testing.

genetic counseling: the process of counseling people who may have a gene that makes them more susceptible to cancer. The purpose of the counseling is to help them decide whether they wish to be tested, to explore what the genetic test results might mean, and to support them before and after the test. *See also* gene, genetic testing, genetic risk factor.

genetic risk factor: a risk factor that is inherited from a parent. A risk factor is anything that increases a person's chance of getting a disease such as cancer. Risk factors can be lifestyle-related or environmental, or genetic (inherited). Having a risk factor, or several risk factors, does not mean that a person will get the disease. Most cancers are not caused by genetic risk factors. If a patient has several family members with cancer, however, genetic testing may be considered. *See also* gene, risk factor, genetic testing, genetic counseling.

genetic testing: tests performed to see if a person has certain gene changes known to increase cancer risk. Such testing is not recommended for everyone, rather for those with specific types of family history. Genetic counseling should be part of the process. *See also* gene, genetic counseling, genetic risk factor.

goiter (GOY-ter): an enlarged thyroid gland. Goiters can be diffuse or nodular and may be caused by insufficient dietary iodine. Although most goiters are not cancerous, they should be evaluated by a physician. A **diffuse goiter** is an enlarged thyroid gland that causes swelling throughout the front part of the neck. A **nodular goiter** is an enlarged thyroid gland caused by a growth or lump that may be benign or malignant.

hematoma (HEE-muh-TOH-muh): a pool of blood, usually clotted, in an organ, tissue, or body space because of a break in the wall of a blood vessel.

hospice: a special kind of care for people in the final phase of illness, their families, and caregivers. The care may take place in the patient's home or in a home-like facility. The focus is on comfort, not cure.

hot nodule: a growth or lump in the thyroid gland that absorbs more radioactivity than the surrounding tissue, as seen during radioiodine scanning. Hot nodules are not usually malignant. *See also* nodule, radioiodine scan, radioactivity. *Compare with* cold nodule.

Hürthle cell carcinoma: Hürthle cell carcinoma of the thyroid gland is an unusual and relatively rare type of differentiated thyroid cancer. Hürthle cells are large and polygonal in shape, with indistinct cell borders. Hürthle cell cancer often is more aggressive than other well-differentiated thyroid cancers. Also called oxyphil cell carcinoma.

hyperplasia: An unusual increase in the number of normal cells in normal arrangement in a tissue or an organ.

hyperplastic: adjectival form of hyperplasia. *See* hyperplasia.

hyperthyroidism (HY-per-THY-ROY-dih-zum): a condition caused by the overproduction of thyroid hormone. Symptoms include weight loss, chest pain, palpitations, diarrhea, nervousness, heat intolerance, and excessive sweating. Also called overactive thyroid. *Compare with* hypothyroidism.

hypothyroidism (HY-poh-THY-ROY-dih-zum): a condition caused by the deficiency of thyroid hormone. Symptoms include weight gain, constipation, dry skin, sensitivity to the cold, fatigue, and lethargy. Also called underactive thyroid. *Compare with* hyperthyroidism.

imaging tests: methods used to produce pictures of internal body structures. Some imaging methods used to help diagnose or stage cancer are x-rays, CT scans, magnetic resonance imaging (MRI), and ultrasound.

informed consent: a legal document that explains a course of treatment, the risks, benefits, and possible alternatives; the process by which patients agree to treatment.

iodine (I-oh-dine): a chemical element necessary for the synthesis of thyroid hormones needed to regulate the metabolic rate in all cells. Dietary iodine can be found in iodized salt and in shell fish.

isthmus: the narrow strip of tissue joining the two lobes of the butterfly–shaped thyroid gland. *See also* lobe, thyroid gland.

lobe: a well-defined portion of an organ such as the brain, lung, liver, breast, or gland.

lobectomy (loh-BEK-toh-mee): the surgical removal of one whole lobe of an organ. *See also* lobe. *Compare with* thyroidectomy.

lymph nodes: small, bean-shaped collections of immune system tissue such as lymphocytes, found along lymphatic vessels. They remove cell waste, germs, and other harmful substances from lymph. They help fight infections and also have a role in fighting cancer, although cancers sometimes spread through lymph nodes. Also called lymph glands.

lymphocyte (LIM-fo-sight): a type of white blood cell that helps the body fight infection.

lymphoma (lim-FOAM-uh): a cancer of the lymphatic system. Lymphoma involves a type of white blood cells called lymphocytes. The 2 main types of lymphoma are Hodgkin disease and non-Hodgkin lymphoma. The treatment methods for these 2 types of lymphomas are very different.

magnetic resonance imaging (MRI): a method of taking pictures of the inside of the body. Instead of using x-rays, MRI uses a powerful magnet to send radio waves through the body. The images appear on a computer screen, as well as on film. Like x-rays, the procedure is physically painless, but some people may feel confined inside the MRI machine, and it is noisy.

malignant: cancerous.

malignant tumor: a mass of cancer cells that may invade surrounding tissues or spread (metastasize) to distant sites in the body. *See also* tumor, metastasis, metastatic cancer.

medullary thyroid carcinoma (MED-yoo-LAYR-ee THY-royd kahr-si-NO-muh): a type of cancer that develops in the C cells of the thyroid gland. The C cells make calcitonin, a hormone that helps maintain a healthy level of calcium in the blood. Medullary thyroid cancer can be either familial (inherited) or sporadic. *See also* familial medullary thyroid carcinoma, C cells, calcitonin, sporadic medullary thyroid cancer.

metabolism: the total of all physical and chemical changes that take place in a cell or an organism. The changes produce energy and materials needed for important life processes.

metastasis (meh-TAS-teh-sis): cancer cells that have spread to one or more sites elsewhere in the body, often by way of the lymphatic system or bloodstream. **Regional metastasis** is cancer that has spread to the lymph nodes, tissues, or organs close to the primary site. **Distant metastasis** is cancer that has spread to organs or tissues that are farther away (such as when colon cancer spreads to the lungs or liver). The plural of this word is metastases. *See also* lymph nodes, metastasize, metastatic.

metastasize (meh-TAS-tuh-size): the spread of cancer cells to one or more sites elsewhere in the body, often by way of the lymphatic system or bloodstream. *See also* metastasis.

metastatic (met-uh-STAT-ick) cancer: a way to describe cancer that has spread from the primary site (where it started) to other structures or organs, nearby or far away (distant). *See also* metastasis, metastasize.

modified radical neck dissection (dye-SEK-shun): surgery to remove all of the lymph nodes located near the thyroid gland and other related tissues in the both in the central portion and along the sides of the neck. *See also* lymph nodes. *Compare with* central compartment neck dissection.

monoclonal (mahn-oh-KLOHN-uhl) antibody: a type of antibody manufactured in the laboratory that is designed to lock onto specific antigens. Antigens are substances that can be recognized by the immune system. Monoclonal antibodies that have been attached to chemotherapy drugs or radioactive substances are being studied for their potential to seek out antigens unique to cancer cells and deliver these treatments directly to the cancer, thus killing the cancer cells and not harming healthy tissue. Monoclonal antibodies are also often used to help detect and classify cancer cells under a microscope. Other studies are being done to see if radioactive atoms attached to monoclonal antibodies can be used in imaging tests to detect and locate small groups of cancer cells. *See* also antibody.

MRI: *see* magnetic resonance imaging.

multiple endocrine neoplasia type 2 (MEN 2), MEN 2a, MEN 2b: a group of rare diseases caused by gene mutations that regulate cell growth leading to hyperplasia and hyperfunction of two or more components of the endocrine system. *See also* hyperplasia.

mutation (myoo-TAY-shun): a permanent change in the DNA of a cell caused by exposure to damaging agents in the environment or mistakes made during cell division (mitosis). Mutations may be harmful, beneficial, or have no effect. Certain mutations may lead to cancer or other disease.

neuroma (NOOR-oh-ma): a tumor growing from a nerve or made up largely of nerve cells and nerve fibers. Many lesions formerly called neuromas are now given more specific names such as ganglioneuroma, neurilenoma, or neurofibroma.

nodule (NOD-yool): a growth or lump in the thyroid gland, often filled with colloid that may be benign or malignant.

octreotide scan: an imaging test using a radioactive drug to detect tumors. Radioactive octreotide is injected into a vein and travels through the bloodstream. Octreotide attaches to tumor cells receptors and can then be identified when a radiation-measuring device detects the location of these tumor cells in the body. *See also* radionuclide scan.

oncogenes: genes that promote cell growth and multiplication. These genes are normally present in all cells. But oncogenes may undergo changes that activate them, causing cells to grow too quickly and form tumors.

oncologist (on-CAHL-uh-jist): a doctor with special training in the diagnosis and treatment of cancer.

oncology: the branch of medicine concerned with the diagnosis and treatment of cancer.

oxyphil cell carcinoma: *see* Hurthle cell carcinoma.

palliation (PA-lee-AY-shun): to relieve or lessen the symptoms and suffering caused by cancer or other life-threatening diseases. The goal of palliation is to improve the patient's quality of life, although it does not cure the disease.

palliative (PA-lee-uh-tiv) treatment: treatment that relieves symptoms, such as pain, but is not expected to cure the disease. Its main purpose is to improve the patient's quality of life. Sometimes chemotherapy and radiation are used as palliative treatments. *Compare with* curative treatment.

papillary adenocarcinoma (PAP-ih-lar-ee A-den-oh-KAR-sih-NOH-muh): a malignant tumor that begins in the epithelial layer (inner lining) of certain internal organs and has gland-like properties. These types of tumors have finger-like processes of vascular connective tissue and occur most frequently in the ovary and thyroid glands.

papillary carcinoma (PAP-ih-lar-ee KAR-sih-NOH-muh): an irregular, solid or cystic cancerous mass that arises from otherwise normal follicular cell tissue in the thyroid. The mass grows in small finger-like shapes and attaches to the epithelial layer (inner lining) of the organ. Papillary tumors are the most common of all thyroid cancers.

papillary thyroid cancer (PA-pih-LAYR-ee THY-royd KAN-ser): *see* papillary carcinoma.

parafollicular cells: *see* C cells.

parathyroid (PAYR-uh-THY-royd) gland: one of four pea-sized glands found on the surface of the thyroid. The parathyroid hormone made by these glands increases the calcium level in the blood.

PET scan: *see* positron emission tomography.

pheochromocytoma (FEE-oh-KROH-moh-sy-TOH-muh): a tumor of special cells (called chromaffin cells) that forms in the center of the adrenal gland, causing the gland to produce too much adrenaline. Pheochromocytomas are usually benign (noncancerous) but are occasionally malignant. These tumors can cause many problems, including high blood pressure, pounding headaches, heart palpitations, flushing of the face, nausea, and vomiting.

pituitary gland (pih-OO-ih-TAYR-ee): a small, oval gland in the base of the brain, which serves as the primary gland in the endocrine system. The secretions of the pituitary gland control the other endocrine glands and influence growth, metabolism, and maturation. *See also* endrocine glands.

positron emission tomography (PAHS-ih-trahn ee-MISH-uhn toh-MAHG-ruh-fee) (PET): a PET scan creates an image of the body (or of biochemical events) after the injection of a very low dose of a radioactive form of a substance such as glucose (sugar). The scan computes the rate at which the tumor is using the sugar. In general, high-grade tumors use more sugar than normal and low-grade tumors use less. PET scans are especially useful in taking images of the brain, although they are becoming more widely used to find the spread of cancer of the breast, colon, rectum, ovary, or lung. PET scans may also be used to see how well the tumor is responding to treatment.

prognosis (prog-NO-sis): a prediction of the course of disease; the outlook for the chances of survival.

quality of life: overall enjoyment of life, which includes a person's sense of well-being and ability to do the things that are important to him or her.

radiation (RAY-dee-AY-shun): energy released in the form of particles or electromagnetic waves. Common sources of radiation include radon gas, cosmic rays from outer space, medical x-rays, and energy given off by a radioisotope.

radiation therapy: treatment with high-energy rays (such as x-rays) to kill or shrink cancer cells. The radiation may come from outside of the body (external radiation) or from radioactive materials placed directly in the tumor (brachytherapy or internal radiation). Radiation therapy may be used as the main treatment for a cancer, to reduce the size of a cancer before surgery, or to destroy any remaining cancer cells after surgery. In advanced cancer cases, it may also be used as palliative treatment. *See also* brachytherapy, external beam radiation therapy, palliative treatment.

radioactive iodine (RAY-dee-oh-AK-tiv I-oh-dine) (RAI): a radioactive form of iodine, often used for imaging tests or to treat an overactive thyroid, thyroid cancer, and certain other cancers. For imaging tests, the patient takes a small dose of radioactive iodine that collects in thyroid cells and certain kinds of tumors and can be detected by a scanner. To treat thyroid cancer, the patient takes a large dose of radioactive iodine, which kills thyroid cells. *See also* iodine, radioiodine scanning, radioiodine therapy.

radioactivity: spontaneous emission of radiation, either directly from unstable atomic nuclei or as a consequence of a nuclear reaction.

radioiodine (RAY-dee-oh-I-oh-dine) scan: the use of low doses of a radioactive form of iodine for imaging tests to detect thyroid cancer. *See also* octreotide scan. *Compare with* radioiodine therapy.

radioiodine (RAY-dee-oh-I-oh-dine) therapy: the use of large doses of a radioactive form of iodine to treat thyroid cancers. Radioactive iodine can be administered by liquid or in capsule form, by infusion, or sealed in seeds placed in or near the tumor designed to destroy the thyroid tissue.

radionuclide scanning (RAY-dee-oh-NOO-klide SKAN-ing): a procedure that uses a special camera to produce pictures (scans) of structures inside the body. Radionuclide scanning is used to diagnose, stage, and monitor disease. During the procedure, a small amount of a chemical substance called an isotope, which exhibits radioactivity, is injected into a vein or swallowed and then travels through the bloodstream to different organs. A computer then forms images of the parts of the body where the radionuclide builds up. These areas may contain cancer cells, but further testing is necessary to confirm the presence of cancer in these areas.

RAI I-131: one form of radioactive iodine. This substance can be used in small doses for cancer detection during radioiodine scanning or in large doses for treating thyroid cancer during radioiodine therapy. *See also* iodine, radioactive iodine, radioiodine scanning, and radioiodine therapy.

recurrence: the return of cancer after treatment. **Local recurrence** means that the cancer has come back at the same place as the original cancer. **Regional recurrence** means that the cancer has come back, after treatment, in the lymph nodes near the primary site. **Distant recurrence,** also known as metastatic recurrence, is when cancer metastasizes, after treatment, to distant organs or tissues (such as the lungs, liver, bone marrow, or brain). *See also* metastasis, metastasize, metastatic.

regional metastasis: *see* metastasis.

risk factor: anything that affects a person's chance of getting a disease such as cancer. Different cancers have different risk factors. For example, unprotected exposure to strong sunlight is a risk factor for skin cancer; smoking is a risk factor for lung, mouth, laryngeal, and other cancers.

Some risk factors, such as smoking, can be controlled. Others, like a person's age, can't be changed.

sentinel lymph node biopsy (BUY-op-see): a diagnostic procedure involving the removal of the first lymph node to which cancer cells are likely to spread from the primary tumor. In some cases, there can be more than one sentinel lymph node. For this procedure, a radioactive substance or contrast dye is injected near the tumor. A scanner is then used to map the circulation of the substance through the primary (sentinel) node. The node is then removed and examined for the presence of cancer cells. *See also* lymph nodes.

side effects: unwanted effects of treatment, such as hair loss caused by chemotherapy and fatigue caused by radiation therapy.

sign: an observable physical change caused by an illness. *Compare with* symptom.

sonogram (SON-o-gram): a computer picture of areas inside the body by the pattern of echoes created by bouncing high-energy sound waves (ultrasound) off internal tissues or organs. Also called an ultrasonogram.

sonography: Sonography is an imaging technique used to visualize soft tissues of the body (muscles and internal organs), their size, structures, and possible pathologies or lesions. Diagnostic sonography is also called ultrasonography.

sporadic medullary thyroid cancer (MED-yoo-LAYR-ee THY-royd KAN-ser): a type of cancer that develops in the C cells of the thyroid gland. C cells make the hormone calcitonin, which helps maintain a healthy level of calcium in the blood. Sporadic cancers are not a result of inherited gene mutations and, occasionally, they occur in a random or isolated manner. *Compare with* familial medullary thyroid cancer.

sporadic MTC: *see* sporadic medullary thyroid cancer.

stage: the extent of a cancer in the body. *See* staging.

staging: the process of finding out whether cancer has spread and, if so, how far. *See* AJCC/TNM systems. The TNM system, which is used most often, gives 3 key pieces of information:

- T refers to the size of the tumor
- N describes how far the cancer has spread to nearby lymph nodes
- M shows whether the cancer has spread (metastasized) to other organs of the body

Letters or numbers after the T, N, and M give more details about each of these factors. To make this information more clear, the TNM descriptions can be grouped together into a simpler set of stages, labeled with Roman numerals (usually from I to IV). In general, the lower the number, the less the cancer has spread. A higher number means a more serious cancer. *See also* pathologic staging, clinical staging.

standard medical treatment: *see* standard therapy.

standard therapy: the most commonly used and widely accepted form of treatment for a disease. *Compare with* unproven therapy.

stromal cell (STROH-mul SEL): a type of cell that makes up certain kinds of connective tissue (supporting tissue that surrounds other tissues and organs).

stromal tumor (STROH-mul): a tumor that arises in the supporting connective tissue of an organ.

symptom: a change in the body caused by an illness, as described by the person experiencing it. *Compare with* sign.

systemic therapy: treatment that reaches and affects cells throughout the entire body, for example, chemotherapy.

thyroglobulin (THY-roh-GLOB-yoo-lin): the stored form of thyroid hormone found only in the cells of the thyroid gland. After a thyroidectomy, thyroglobulin should no longer show up on a blood test. Since thyroglobulin is normally only made by thyroid cells, it can serve as a tumor marker to indicate remaining thyroid cells after the treatment. *See also* thyroidectomy.

thyroid capsule (THY-royd KAP-sool): the sac of tissue and blood vessels that surrounds the thyroid gland.

thyroidectomy (THY-roy-DEK-toh-mee): a surgical procedure to remove part or all of the thyroid gland.

thyroid follicular cell (THY-royd fuh-LIH-kyoo-ler sel): the hormone-producing cell(s) in the thyroid gland.

thyroid (THY-royd) gland: the butterfly-shaped gland that produces thyroid hormone. The thyroid gland is located beneath the voice box (larynx) and is part of the endocrine system. It is essential to normal body growth in infancy and childhood and regulates the metabolic rate in adults. In addition, the thyroid gland influences body processes like growth, development, and reproduction.

thyroid lymphoma: a form of cancer that develops from white blood cells called lymphocytes. Lymphocytes are normally present in the thyroid gland. *See also* lymphocytes. Through a process of transformation, these white blood cells may start to grow abnormally, expanding to form a mass called a lymphoma. This mass can grow rapidly and may expand to the point where it compresses other structures in the neck, causing problems with speech, swallowing, or breathing. Thyroid lymphoma usually responds well to treatment with external beam radiation therapy and chemotherapy.

thyroid nodules: *see* nodule.

thyroid sarcoma: an aggressive tumor that develops in the stromal or vascular tissue in the thyroid gland. Sarcomas that arise in the thyroid gland are uncommon. The treatment for thyroid sarcomas is total thyroidectomy. Radiation therapy may be used in addition to surgery. Most sarcomas are unresponsive to chemotherapy. Recurrence is common, as it is with sarcomas arising in other sites in the body, and the patient's overall prognosis is poor.

thyroid-stimulating hormone (TSH): a hormone, also known as thyrotropin, released by the pituitary gland that stimulates the thyroid gland to produce hormones that regulate metabolism.

thyrotropin: a synthetic (man-made) form of thyroid-stimulating hormone (TSH) used to detect remaining or recurring cancer cells in patients who have received treatment for thyroid cancer.

tissue: a collection of cells, united to perform a particular function in the body.

TNM staging system: *see* staging.

tracheostomy (TRAY-kee-OS-toh-mee): surgical construction of a opening (stoma) in the trachea (windpipe) to assist with respiration. The stoma may also be referred to as a tracheostomy.

transducer: a device that converts one form of energy, such as pressure, temperature, or pulse, into another form of energy, often an electrical signal.

TSH: *see* thyroid-stimulating hormone.

tumor: an abnormal lump or mass of tissue. Tumors can be benign (noncancerous) or malignant (cancerous).

tumor suppressor genes: genes that slow down cell division or cause cells to die at the appropriate time. Alterations of these genes can lead to too much cell growth and development of cancer.

tyrosine kinase inhibitor: a drug that interferes with cell communication and growth and may prevent tumor growth. Some tyrosine kinase inhibitors are used to treat cancer.

ultrasound: an imaging method in which high-frequency sound waves are used to outline a part of the body. The sound wave echoes are picked up and displayed on a screen. Also called ultrasonography. *See also* sonogram.

undifferentiated cells: cells that bear little resemblance to healthy organ tissue cells. Undifferentiated cancer cells (also called anaplastic carcinomas) are more likely to be aggressive cancers. *Compare with* differentiated cells.

unproven therapy: any therapy that has not been scientifically tested and approved. *Compare with* standard therapy.

U.S. Food and Drug Administration (FDA): an agency of the United States Department of Health and Human Services. The FDA is responsible for regulating drugs, biological medical products, blood products, medical devices, and radiation-emitting devices, along with other products.

x-ray: one form of radiation that can be used at low levels to produce an image of the body on film or at high levels to destroy cancer cells.

Index

Books Published
by the American Cancer Society

Available everywhere books are sold and online at
www.cancer.org/bookstore

Information

American Cancer Society's Complete Guide to Colorectal Cancer

American Cancer Society's Complete Guide to Prostate Cancer

Breast Cancer Clear & Simple: All Your Questions Answered

The Cancer Atlas (available in English, Spanish, French, and Chinese)

Cancer: What Causes It, What Doesn't

QuickFACTS™ - Advanced Cancer

QuickFACTS™ - Bone Metastasis

QuickFACTS™ - Colorectal Cancer, Second Edition

QuickFACTS™ - Lung Cancer

QuickFACTS™ - Prostate Cancer

The Tobacco Atlas, Second Edition (available in English, Spanish and French)

Day-to-Day Help

American Cancer Society's Guide to Pain Control: Understanding and Managing Cancer Pain, Revised Edition

Cancer Caregiving A to Z: An At-Home Guide for Patients and Families

Caregiving: A Step-By-Step Resource for Caring for the Person with Cancer at Home, Revised Edition

Eating Well, Staying Well During and After Cancer

Get Better! Communication Cards for Kids & Adults

Lymphedema: Understanding and Managing Lymphedema After Cancer Treatment

Social Work in Oncology: Supporting Survivors, Families and Caregivers

When the Focus Is on Care: Palliative Care and Cancer

Emotional Support

Angels & Monsters: A child's eye view of cancer

Cancer in the Family: Helping Children Cope with a Parent's Illness

Couples Confronting Cancer: Keeping Your Relationship Strong

Crossing Divides: A Couple's Story of Cancer, Hope, and Hiking Montana's Continental Divide

I Can Survive

What Helped Get Me Through: Cancer Survivors Share Wisdom and Hope

Just for Kids

Because . . . Someone I Love Has Cancer: Kids' Activity Book

Healthy Me: A Read-Along Coloring & Activity Book

Kids' First Cookbook: Delicious-Nutritious Treats To Make Yourself!

Mom and the Polka-Dot Boo-Boo

Our Dad Is Getting Better

Our Mom Has Cancer (hardcover)

Our Mom Has Cancer (paperback)

Our Mom Is Getting Better

Prevention

The American Cancer Society's Healthy Eating Cookbook: A celebration of food, friendship, and healthy living, Third Edition

Celebrate! Healthy Entertaining for Any Occasion

Good for You! Reducing Your Risk of Developing Cancer

The Great American Eat-Right Cookbook: 140 Great-Tasting, Good-for-You Recipes

Healthy Air: A Read-Along Coloring & Activity Book (25 per pack: Tobacco avoidance)

Healthy Bodies: A Read-Along Coloring & Activity Book (25 per pack: Physical activity)

Healthy Food: A Read-Along Coloring & Activity Book (25 per pack: Nutrition)

Kicking Butts: Quit Smoking and Take Charge of Your Health

National Health Education Standards: Achieving Excellence, Second Edition (available in paperback and on CD-ROM)

DATE DUE

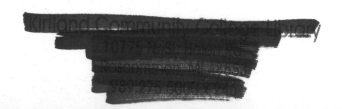

Kirtland Community College Library
10775 N. St. Helen Rd.
Roscommon, MI 48653
989-275-5000 EXT 246